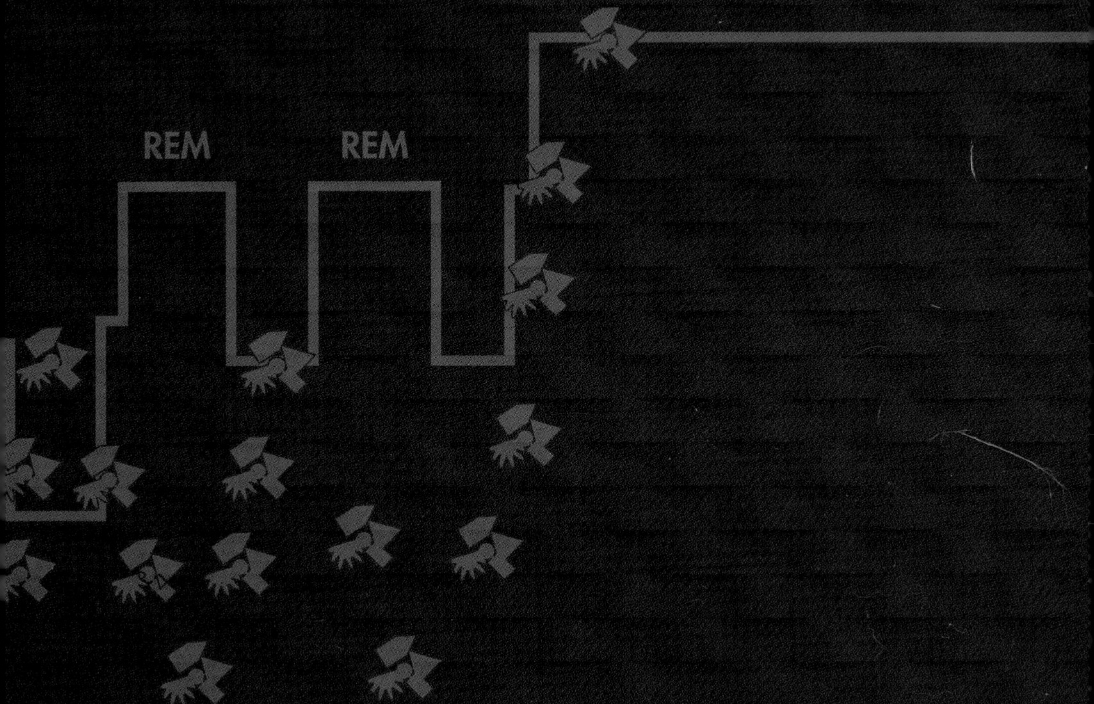

WAKING THE BRAIN:

An Update on the Neurobiology, Diagnosis, and Treatment of Hypersomnia

Every effort has been made in preparing this book to provide accurate and up-to-date information that is in accord with accepted standards and practice at the time of publication. Nevertheless, the author, editors, and publisher can make no warranties that the information contained herein is totally free from error, not least because clinical standards are constantly changing through research and regulation. The author, editors, and publisher therefore disclaim all liability for direct or consequential damages resulting from the use of material contained in this book. Readers are strongly advised to pay careful attention to information provided by the manufacturer of any drugs or equipment that they plan to use.

PUBLISHED BY NEI PRESS, an imprint of NEUROSCIENCE EDUCATION INSTITUTE
Carlsbad, California, United States of America
NEUROSCIENCE EDUCATION INSTITUTE
1930 Palomar Point Way, Suite 101
Carlsbad, California 92008

http://www.neiglobal.com

Printed in the United States of America
First Edition, October 2015

Typeset in Myriad Pro

Library of Congress Cataloging-in-Publication Data
ISBN 978-1-4225-0098-5

Table of Contents

CME Information

Overview

Although there is still much debate over the exact function of sleep, in the past decade, our understanding of the molecular and biological processes that underlie sleep and wake states has increased exponentially. We have also become more aware of the physiological and psychiatric consequences of disturbed sleep. In this book, we provide an update on the current knowledge of the environmental, neurobiological, and genetic factors that influence sleep and wakefulness. We also provide evidence-based guidance for the accurate diagnosis and optimal treatment of disorders of hypersomnolence.

Target Audience

This activity has been developed for prescribers specializing in psychiatry. All other health care providers interested in psychopharmacology are welcome for advanced study, especially primary care physicians, nurse practitioners, psychologists, and pharmacists.

Statement of Need

Narcolepsy is a debilitating neurodegenerative disorder characterized by excessive sleepiness and rapid eye movement (REM) sleep abnormalities. The disorder can have deleterious effects on physical and mental health as well as on functioning and work productivity. Documented health consequences include increased risk of hypercholesterolemia, digestive diseases, heart disease, and hypertension as well as increased risk of major depression and anxiety disorders.

- The lack of knowledge about narcolepsy among physicians indicates a need for education in this area, particularly since sleep medicine is an evolving field that has experienced significant strides in recent years.
- Continuing education on narcolepsy and the medications used to treat it is essential in order for clinicians to implement best practices for its management in clinical practice.

To help address clinician performance deficits with respect to sleep/wake disorders, quality improvement efforts need to provide education regarding 1) updating knowledge on our current understanding of the neurobiological bases of narcolepsy; 2) applying evidence-based practice guidelines to the accurate identification and diagnosis of narcolepsy; and 3) implementing pharmacological and nonpharmacological treatment strategies tailored to the needs of the individual patient.

Learning Objectives

After completing the activity, you should be better able to:

- Review the neurobiological and molecular bases of sleep-wake cycles
- Implement the diagnostic assessment of patients with hypersomnia according to established best practices
- Optimize treatment strategies to address hypersomnia in patients with sleep/wake disorders

Accreditation and Credit Designation Statements

The Neuroscience Education Institute is accredited by the Accreditation Council for Continuing Medical Education (ACCME) to provide continuing medical education for physicians.

The Neuroscience Education Institute designates this enduring material for a maximum of 2.5 *AMA PRA Category 1 Credits*™. Physicians should claim only the credit commensurate with the extent of their participation in the activity.

The American Society for the Advancement of Pharmacotherapy (ASAP), Division 55 of the American Psychological Association, is approved by the American Psychological Association to sponsor continuing education for psychologists. ASAP maintains responsibility for this program and its content.

The American Society for the Advancement of Pharmacotherapy designates this program for 2.5 CE credits for psychologists.

Nurses: for all of your CNE requirements for recertification, the ANCC will accept *AMA PRA Category 1 Credits*™ from organizations accredited by the ACCME. The content of this activity pertains to pharmacology and is worth 2.5 continuing education hours of pharmacotherapeutics.

Physician Assistants: the NCCPA accepts *AMA PRA Category 1 Credits*™ from organizations accredited by the AMA (providers accredited by the ACCME).

A certificate of participation for completing this activity is available.

Note: the content of this print monograph activity also exists as an electronic book under the same title. If you received CME credit for the electronic book version, you will not be able to receive credit again for completing this print monograph version.

Optional Posttest and CME Credit Instructions

The estimated time for completion of this activity is 2.5 hours. There is no posttest fee nor fee for CME credits.

1. Read the book in sequence, evaluating the content presented
2. Complete the posttest and activity evaluation, available only online at www.neiglobal.com/CME (under "Book")
3. Print your certificate (if a score of 70% or more is achieved)
4. Questions? call 888-535-5600, or email CustomerService@NEIglobal.com

Peer Review

This material has been peer-reviewed by an MD to ensure the scientific accuracy and medical relevance of information presented and its independence from commercial bias. The Neuroscience Education Institute takes responsibility for the content, quality, and scientific integrity of this CME activity.

Disclosures

It is the policy of NEI to ensure balance, independence, objectivity, and scientific rigor in all its educational activities. Therefore, all individuals in a position to influence or control content are required to disclose any financial relationships. Although potential conflicts of interest are identified and resolved prior to the activity being presented, it remains for the participant to determine whether outside interests reflect a possible bias in either the exposition or the conclusions presented.

Disclosed financial relationships with conflicts of interest have been reviewed by the NEI CME Advisory Board Chair and resolved.

Author/Developer
Debbi Ann Morrissette, PhD
Adjunct Professor, Biological Sciences, Palomar College, San Marcos, CA
Senior Medical Writer, Neuroscience Education Institute, Carlsbad, CA
No financial relationships to disclose.

Content Editor
Stephen M. Stahl, MD, PhD
Adjunct Professor, Department of Psychiatry, University of California, San Diego School of Medicine, San Diego, CA
Honorary Visiting Senior Fellow, University of Cambridge, UK
Director of Psychopharmacology, California Department of State Hospitals, Sacramento, CA
Grant/Research: Alkermes, Clintara, Forest, Forum, Genomind, JayMac, Jazz, Lilly, Merck, Novartis, Otsuka America, Pamlab, Pfizer, Servier, Shire, Sprout, Sunovion, Sunovion UK, Takeda, Teva, Tonix
Consultant/Advisor: Acadia, BioMarin, Forum/EnVivo, Jazz, Orexigen, Otsuka America, Pamlab, Servier, Shire, Sprout, Taisho, Takeda, Trius
Speakers Bureau: Forum, Servier, Sunovion UK, Takeda
Board Member: BioMarin, Forum/EnVivo, Genomind, Lundbeck, Otsuka America, RCT Logic, Shire

The **Peer Reviewer**, **Design Staff**, and **Planning Committee** have no financial relationships to disclose.

Disclosure of Off-Label Use

This educational activity may include discussion of unlabeled and/or investigational uses of agents that are not currently labeled for such use by the FDA. Please consult the product prescribing information for full disclosure of labeled uses.

Disclaimer

Participants have an implied responsibility to use the newly acquired information from this activity to enhance patient outcomes and their own professional development. The information presented in this educational activity is not meant to serve as a guideline for patient management. Any procedures, medications, or other courses of diagnosis or treatment discussed or suggested in this educational activity should not be used by clinicians without evaluation of their patients' conditions and possible contraindications or dangers in use, review of any applicable manufacturer's product information, and comparison with recommendations of other authorities. Primary references and full prescribing information should be consulted.

Cultural and Linguistic Competency

A variety of resources addressing cultural and linguistic competency can be found at this link: nei.global/CMEregs

Provider

This activity is provided by the Neuroscience Education Institute.

Additionally provided by the American Society for the Advancement of Pharmacotherapy.

Support

This activity is supported by an unrestricted educational grant from Jazz Pharmaceuticals, Inc.

Date of Release/Expiration

Print Monograph Released: October, 2015

Electronic Books Released: October, 2015

CME Credit Expires: October, 2018

Objectives

1. Review the neurobiological and molecular bases of the sleep/wake cycles

2. Implement the diagnostic assessment of patients with hypersomnia according to established best practices

3. Optimize treatment strategies to address hypersomnia in patients with sleep/wake disorders

Introduction

Sleep was once described as a vital behavior of unknown function (Roth and Roehrs, 2000). Although there is still much debate over the exact function of sleep, in the past decade, our understanding of the molecular and biological processes that underlie sleep and wake states has increased exponentially. We have also become more aware of the physiological and psychiatric consequences of disturbed sleep. In this book, we provide an update on the current knowledge of the environmental, neurobiological, and genetic factors that influence sleep and wakefulness. We also provide evidence-based guidance for the accurate diagnosis and optimal treatment of disorders of hypersomnolence.

1

Neurobiological and Molecular Bases of the Sleep/Wake Cycle

Chapter 1 seeks to convey the importance of sleep to whole body wellness. In this chapter, we discuss the sleep/wake cycle and how this circadian behavior is affected by a myriad of neurotransmitter systems. We also discuss the molecular clock, a series of interacting transcription factors that influence sleep and many other physiological processes, and how genetic variation in molecular clock components may influence the sleep/wake cycle as well as cardiometabolic health, mental illness propensity, and risk of cancer. In gaining a deeper understanding of the neurobiological and molecular bases of the sleep/wake cycle, clinicians should be better able to understand the tools used to make a differential diagnosis in patients who present with disorders of hypersomnolence and implement optimal treatment strategies for patients by appreciating the mechanisms by which various agents may affect the sleep/wake cycle.

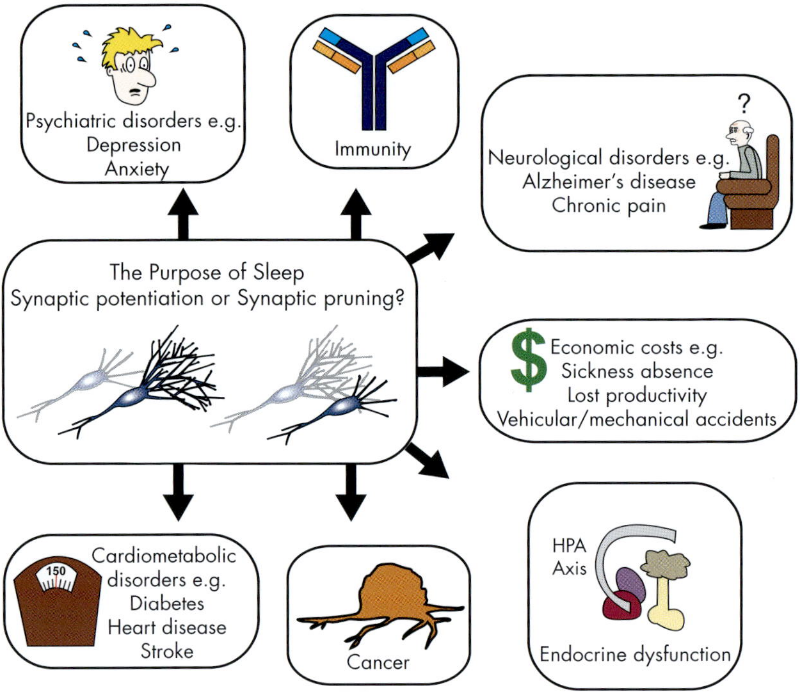

FIGURE 1.1. There is still much debate over the purpose of sleep. Some propose that sleep is essential for synaptic growth, while others argue that sleep is necessary for synaptic pruning (Mignot, 2012; Dresler et al., 2014). Regardless of which hypothesis (or some combination of both) is more accurate, it has become increasingly evident that disturbances of the sleep/wake cycle have a detrimental effect on a myriad of physiological and psychiatric functions. Aside from the economic costs of sleep/wake disorders, the risk of cardiometabolic disease, cancer, mental illness, and overall poorer quality of life are all increased when the sleep/wake cycle is disturbed (Cappuccio et al., 2010; Gui et al., 2013; Lallukka et al., 2014; Liu et al., 2013; Ohayon, 2012; Palma et al., 2013; Pigeon et al., 2012).

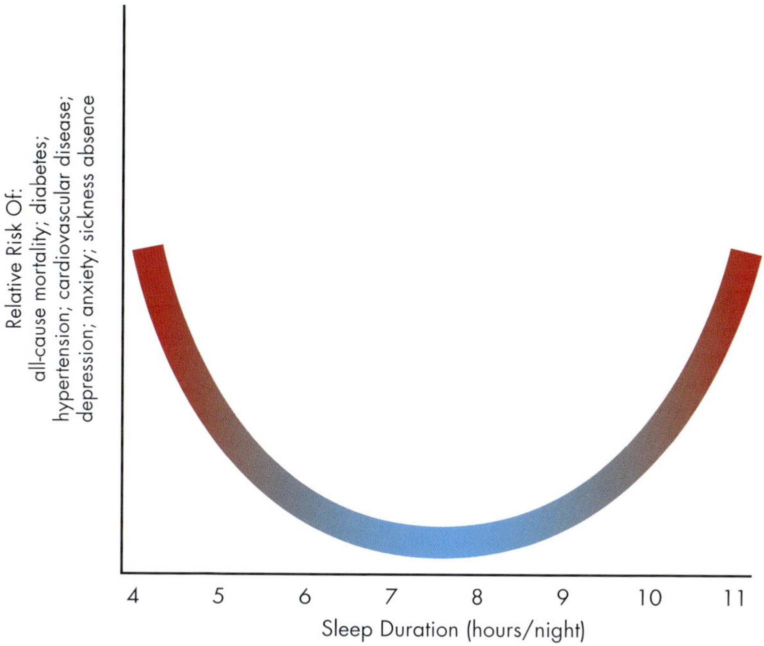

FIGURE 1.2. Both a short duration (<7 hours/night) and a long duration (>9 hours/night) of sleep have been associated with a variety of physiological and psychiatric illnesses, such as diabetes and depression, as well as an increased risk of death (Cappuccio et al., 2010; Guo et al., 2013; Lallukka et al., 2014; Liu et al., 2013). These data, represented here as a U-shaped curve, highlight the notion of the sleep/wake cycle as a homeostatic process that requires a careful balance in order to maintain optimal health.

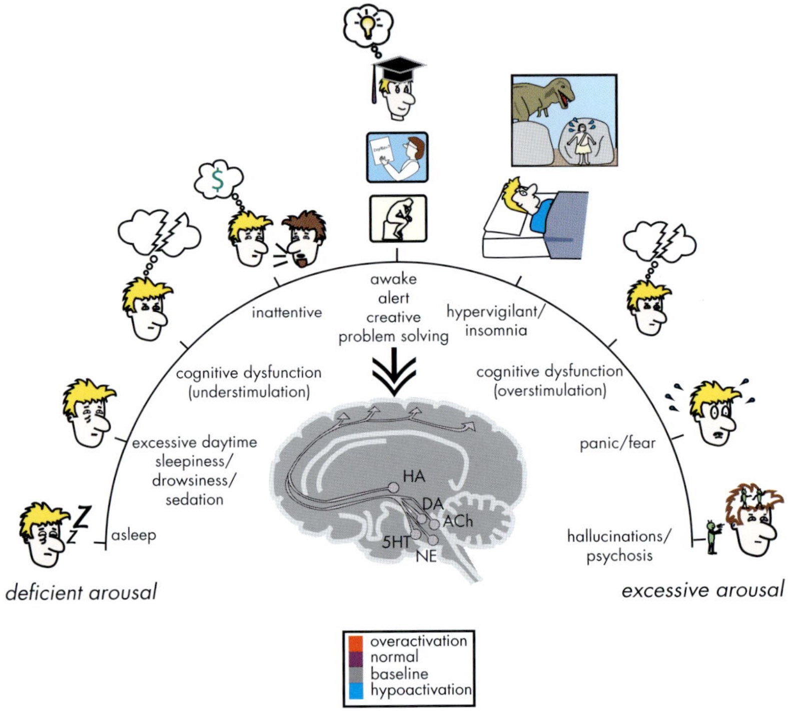

FIGURE 1.3. One's state of arousal is more complicated than simply being awake or asleep. Arousal exists as if on a dimmer switch, with many phases along the spectrum. Where on the spectrum one lies is influenced in large part by 5 key neurotransmitters: histamine, dopamine, norepinephrine, serotonin, and acetylcholine. When there is balance between too much and too little arousal [depicted here by the gray (baseline) color of the brain], one is awake, alert, and able to function well. As the dial shifts to the right, there is too much arousal, which may cause hypervigilance and consequently insomnia at night. Further increases in arousal can cause cognitive dysfunction, panic, and in extreme cases hallucinations. On the other hand, as arousal diminishes, individuals may experience inattentiveness, cognitive dysfunction, sleepiness, and ultimately sleep (Stahl, 2013).

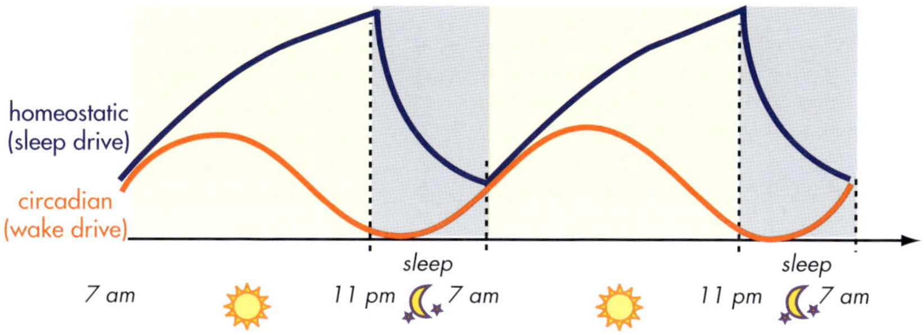

FIGURE 1.4. The sleep/wake cycle is mediated by 2 opposing drives: the homeostatic sleep drive and the circadian wake drive. The homeostatic drive accumulates throughout periods of wakefulness and is opposed by the circadian drive. The longer an individual is awake, the greater the homeostatic drive (Krystal et al., 2010). This homeostatic drive is dependent upon the accumulation of adenosine, which leads to the disinhibition of the ventrolateral preoptic (VLPO) nucleus and the release of GABA/galanin as part of the sleep circuit. The circadian drive, mediated by light acting upon the suprachiasmatic nucleus (SCN), stimulates the release of hypocretin/orexin as part of the wake circuit (Wulff et al., 2010).

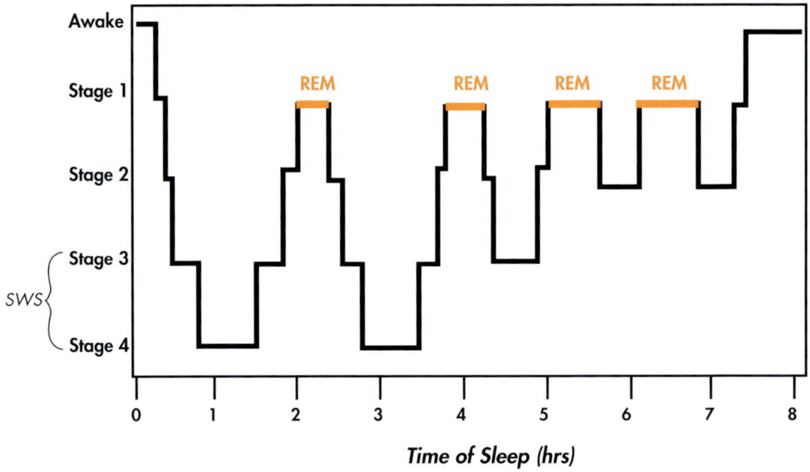

FIGURE 1.5. The complete sleep cycle (non-REM and REM) lasts approximately 90 minutes and occurs 4 to 5 times a night (Reeve and Bailes, 2010). Stages 1 and 2 comprise light non-REM sleep, whereas stages 3 and 4 are part of deeper, slow-wave sleep (SWS) (Tafti, 2009). During the normal sleep period, the duration of non-REM sleep is gradually reduced while the duration of REM sleep is increased. REM sleep is characterized by faster activity on an electroencephalogram (EEG)—similar to that seen during periods of wakefulness—as well as distinct eye movements and peripheral muscle atonia. It is during REM sleep that dreaming occurs, and PET studies have shown activation of the thalamus, the visual cortex, and limbic regions accompanied by reduced metabolism in other regions, such as the dorsolateral prefrontal cortex (DLPFC) and the parietal cortex, during REM sleep. In contrast, there is overall reduced brain activity during non-REM sleep (Larson-Prior et al., 2014).

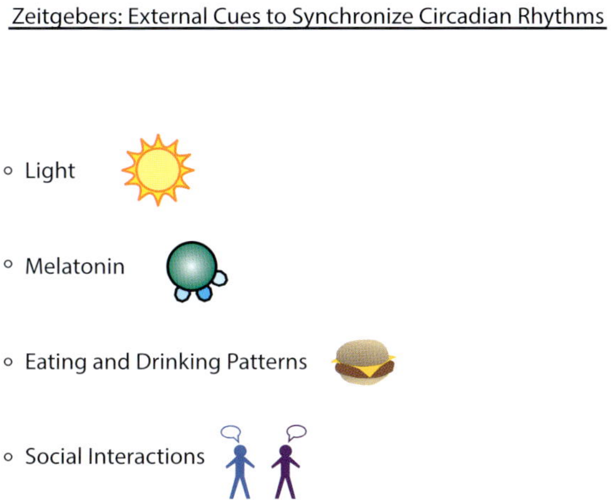

FIGURE 1.6. Virtually all living creatures have an internal molecular clock that synchronizes biological processes such as the sleep/wake cycle and metabolism to a 24-hour circadian rhythm. Although the molecular clock is self-sustaining, it needs to be reset daily. If the molecular clock is not reset, it will drift and become out of sync with environmental cues. These synchronizing cues, termed zeitgebers, include light/dark cycles generated by the movement of the Earth, endogenous or exogenous melatonin, social interactions, and food availability (Van Someren et al., 2007).

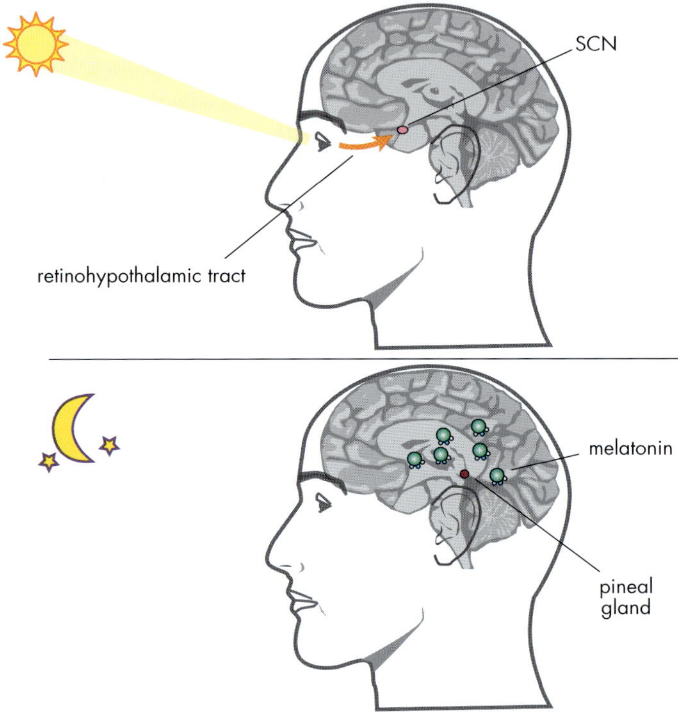

FIGURE 1.7. Although various factors can reset the clock, light is the most powerful synchronizer. When light enters through the eye, it is tranferred via the retinohypothalamic tract to the suprachiasmatic nucleus (SCN) within the hypothalamus. During periods of darkness, the SCN induces the release of melatonin from the pineal gland whereas light suppresses the release of melatonin (Zawilska, 2009).

Control of Sleep By The Suprachiasmatic Nucleus

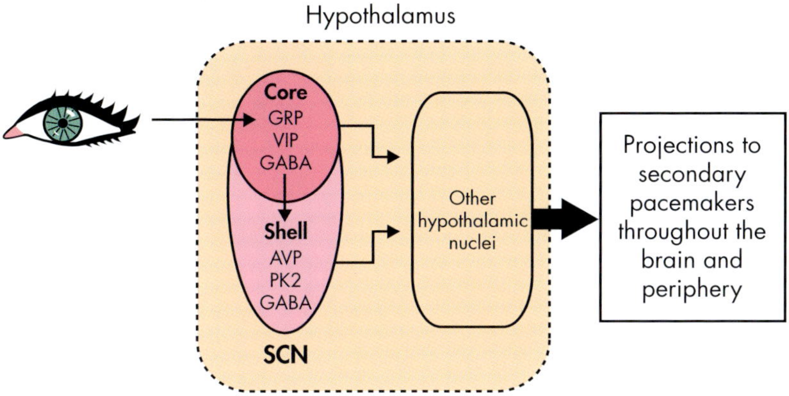

FIGURE 1.8. The main circadian pacemaker is the suprachiasmatic nucleus (SCN), which is located in the hypothalamus. The hypothalamus coordinates the secondary oscillators that are located throughout the periphery and that control many physiological functions, including metabolism, hormone secretion, and cell division. The SCN consists of 2 primary subregions: a ventrolateral core and a dorsomedial shell. The core contains neurons that release the neuropeptides vasoactive intestinal peptide (VIP) and gastrin-releasing peptide (GRP) as well as the neurotransmitter GABA. The core receives the majority of the light coming through the retinohypothalamic tract (as well as input from other brain regions) and utilizes this information to synchronize the SCN with light/dark cycles. The shell of the SCN contains neurons that release arginine-vasopressin (AVP), prokineticin 2 (PK2), and GABA. These neurons receive input from the SCN core and use this information to synchronize the SCN with peripheral oscillators (Brancaccio et al., 2014; Colwell, 2011).

Brain Regions Involved in the Sleep/Wake Cycle

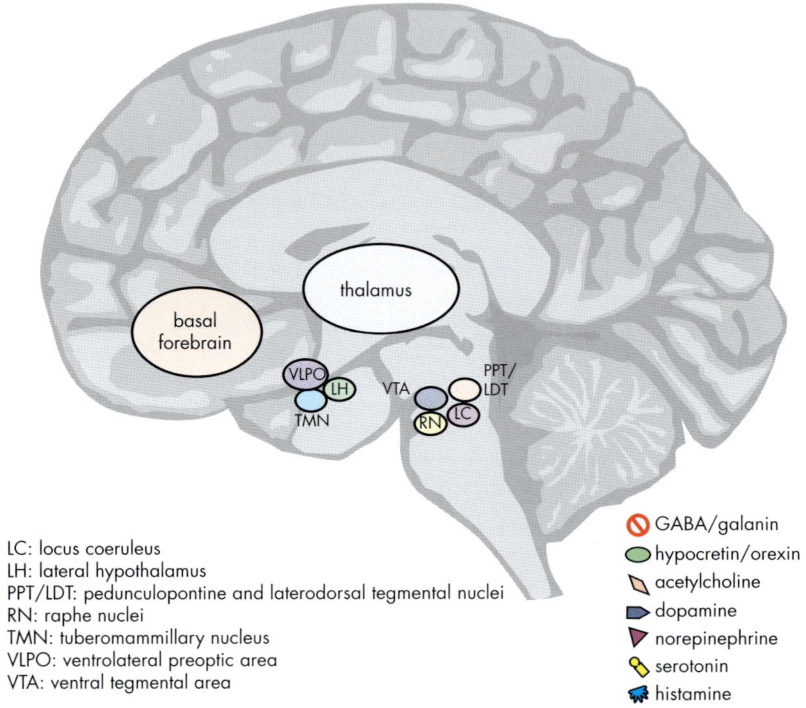

FIGURE 1.9. The sleep/wake cycle is maintained by a series of sleep-promoting and wake-promoting circuits located throughout the brain. Utilizing a variety of neurotransmitter and neuropeptide molecules, these circuits modulate one another via an intricate series of interacting loops.

The Sleep Circuit

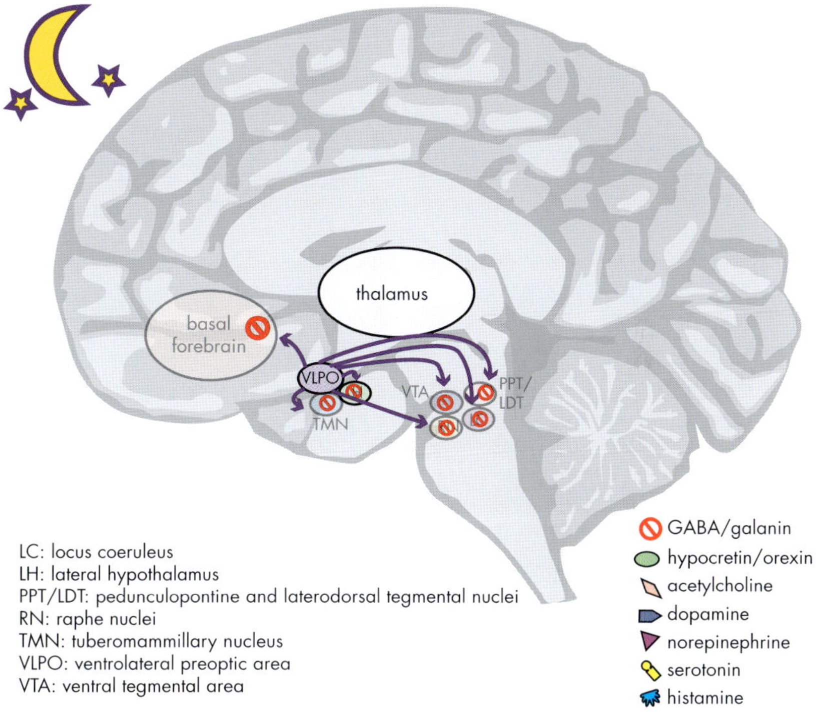

FIGURE 1.10. The sleep circuit is dependent upon the release of GABA and galanin from the ventrolateral preoptic (VLPO) nucleus of the hypothalamus. During periods of darkness, GABAergic projections from the VLPO nucleus inhibit activity in brain regions of the wake-promoting circuit, including the tuberomammillary nucleus (TMN), the lateral hypothalamus (LH), the basal forebrain (BF), the pedunculopontine and laterodorsal tegmental (PPT/LDT) nuclei, the ventral tegmental area (VTA), the locus coeruleus (LC), and the raphe nucleus (RN).

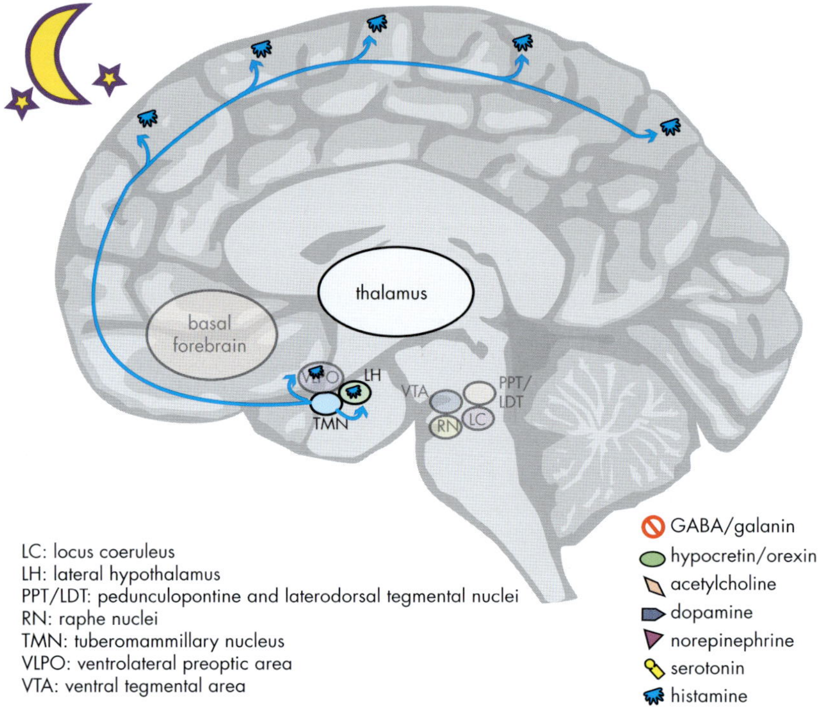

FIGURE 1.11. During periods of light, histamine is released from the tuberomammillary nucleus onto neurons throughout the cortex and in the ventrolateral preoptic area, inhibiting the release of GABA.

The Wake Circuit: Part 2

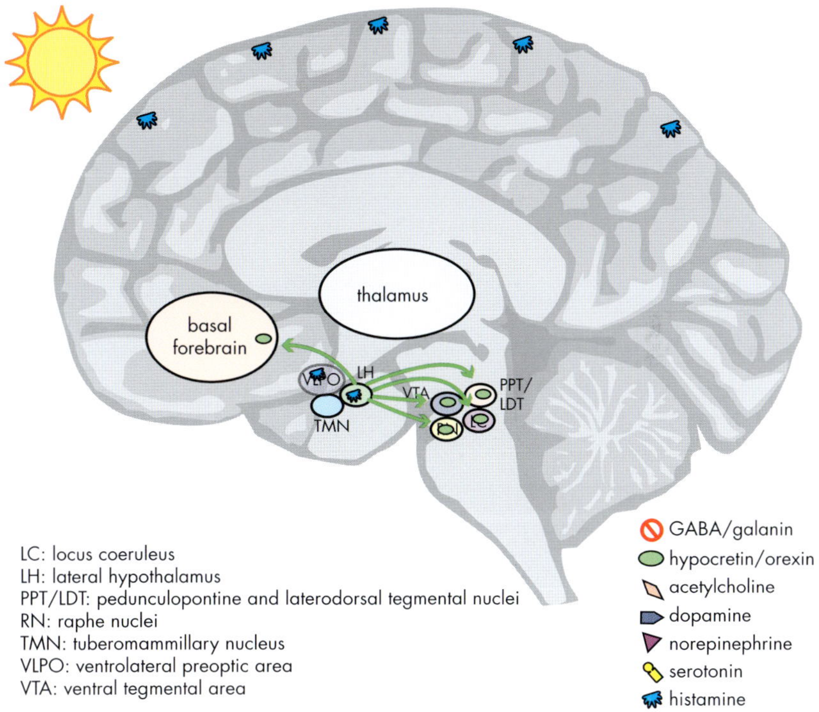

FIGURE 1.12. Histamine from the tuberomammillary nucleus also stimulates the release of hypocretin, also known as orexin, from the lateral hypothalamus. Hypocretin in turn activates other elements of the wake-promoting circuit.

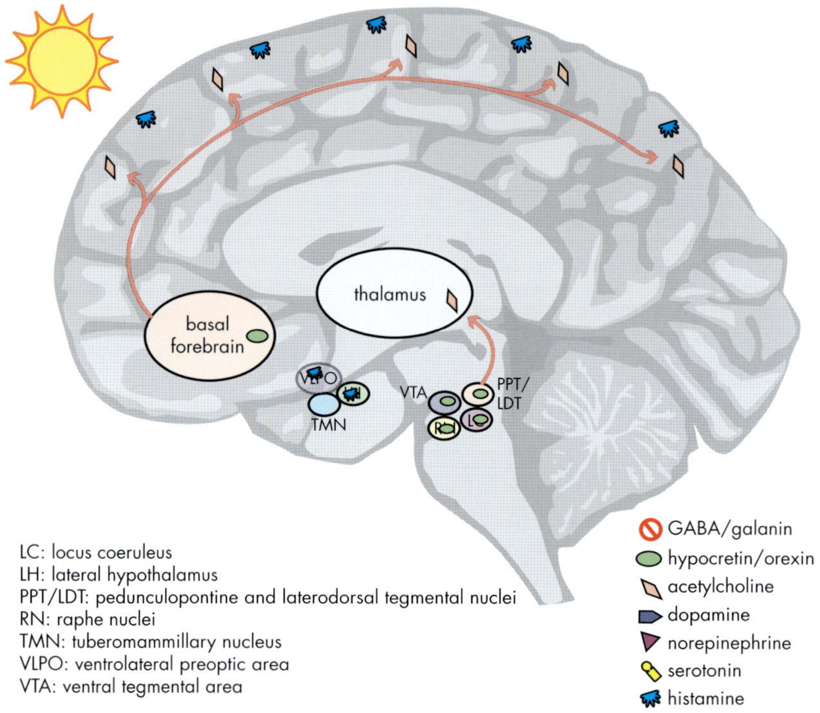

FIGURE 1.13. Hypocretin/orexin induces the release of acetylcholine from the basal forebrain in cortical areas and the release of acetylcholine from the pedunculopontine and laterodorsal tegmental nuclei onto the thalamus.

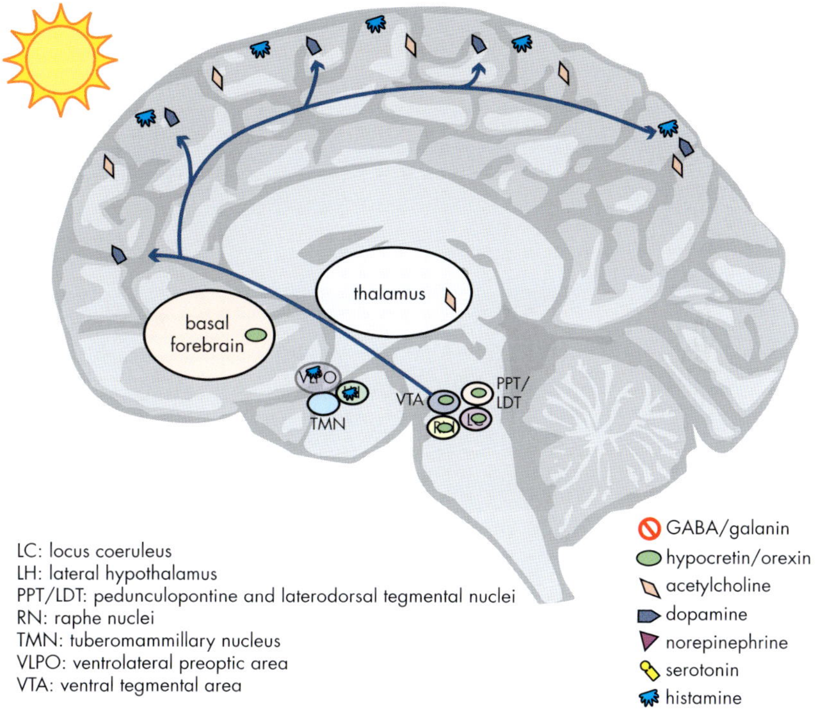

FIGURE 1.14. Hypocretin/orexin also causes the release of dopamine from the ventral tegmental area onto cortical areas.

The Wake Circuit: Part 5

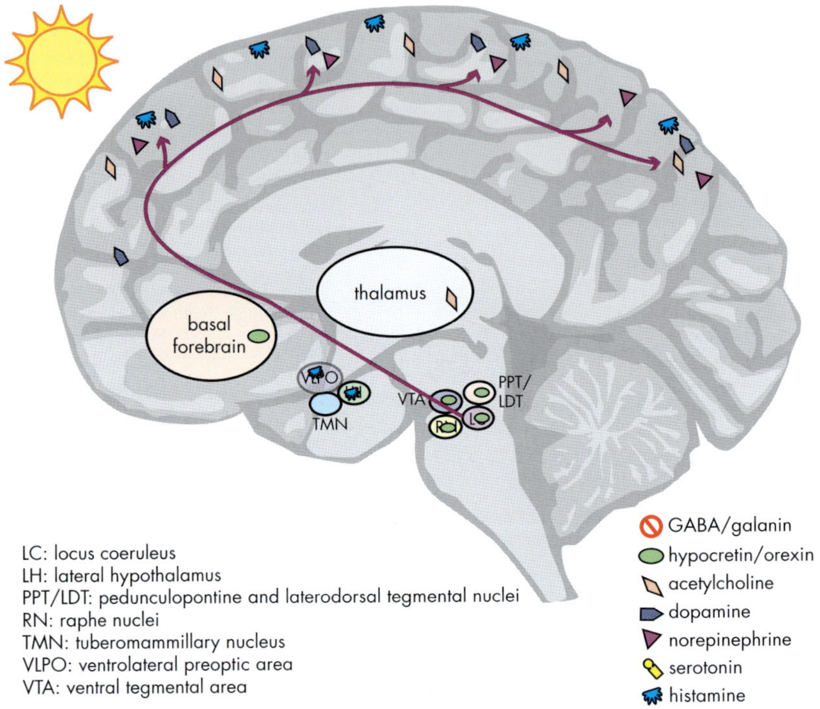

FIGURE 1.15. Additionally, hypocretin/orexin stimulates the release of norepinephrine from the locus coeruleus onto cortical areas.

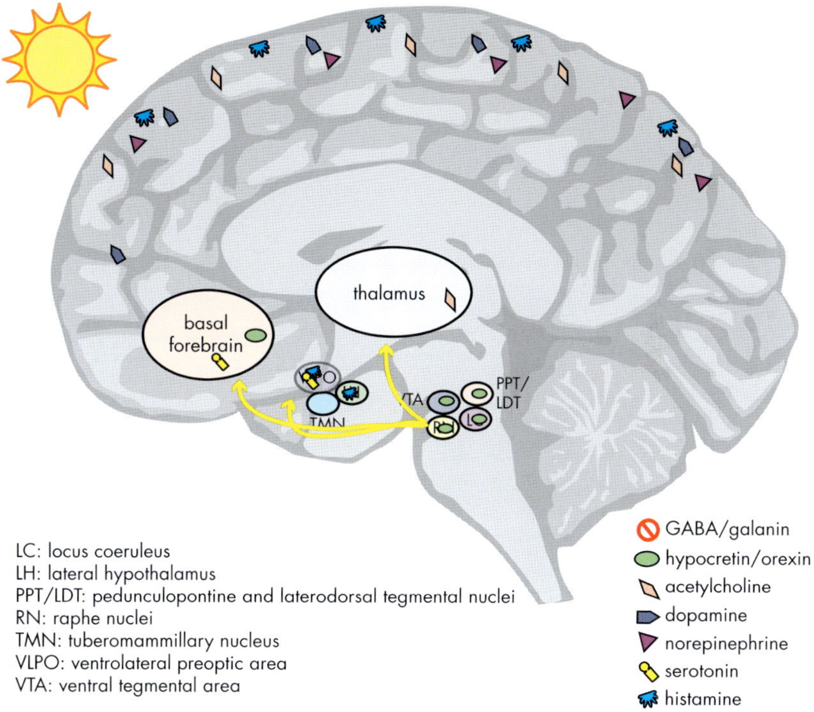

FIGURE 1.16. Hypocretin/orexin also instigates the release of serotonin from the raphe nucleus onto both the basal forebrain and the thalamus.

Triggering the Sleep Circuit

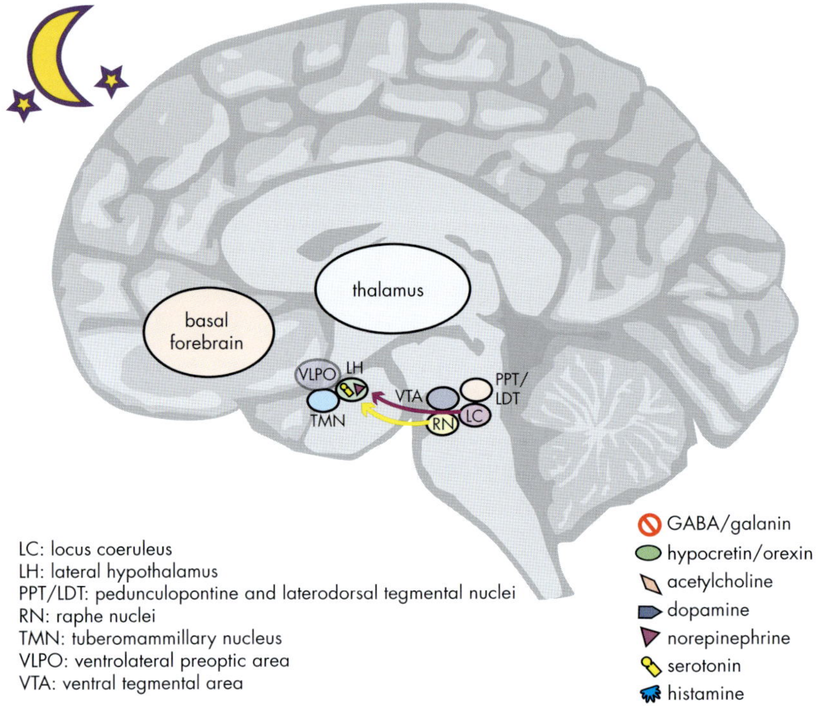

FIGURE 1.17. Furthermore, norepinephrine from the locus coeruleus and serotonin from the raphe nucleus are released onto neurons in the lateral hypothalamus, inhibiting the release of hypocretin.

Without hypocretin/orexin, the ventrolateral preoptic nucleus is disinhibited. The activated ventrolateral preoptic nucleus therefore releases GABA and galanin, inhibiting wake circuitry and initiating the sleep circuit.

Neurotransmitter Levels Throughout the Sleep/Wake Cycle: GABA/Galanin

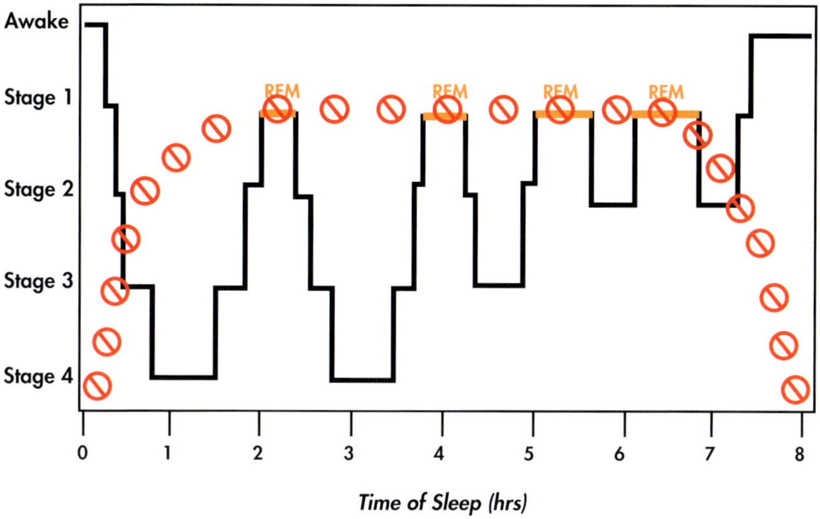

FIGURE 1.18. Neurotransmitters fluctuate not only on a circadian (24-hour) basis, but also throughout the sleep cycle. GABA and galanin levels steadily increase during the first couple of hours of sleep, plateau, and then steadily decline before one wakes.

Neurotransmitter Levels Throughout the Sleep/Wake Cycle: Hypocretin/Orexin

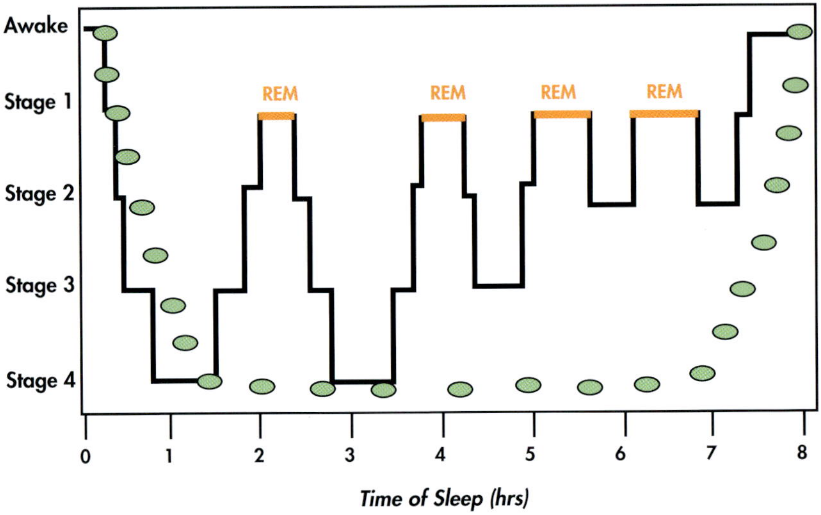

FIGURE 1.19. Unlike GABA/galanin, hypocretin/orexin levels steadily decrease during the first couple of hours of sleep, plateau, and then steadily increase before one wakes.

Neurotransmitter Levels Throughout the Sleep/Wake Cycle: Acetylcholine

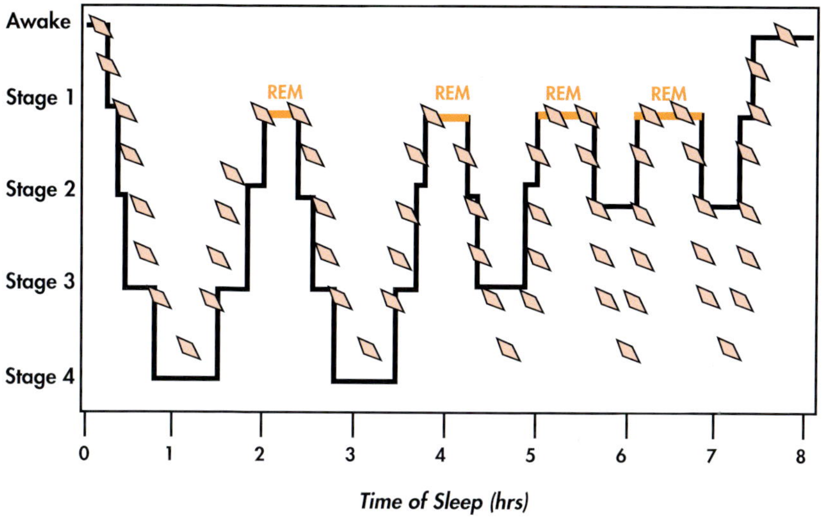

FIGURE 1.20. Acetylcholine levels fluctuate throughout the sleep cycle, reaching their lowest levels during stage 4 sleep and peaking during REM sleep.

Neurotransmitter Levels Throughout the Sleep/Wake Cycle: Dopamine, Norepinephrine, Serotonin, and Histamine

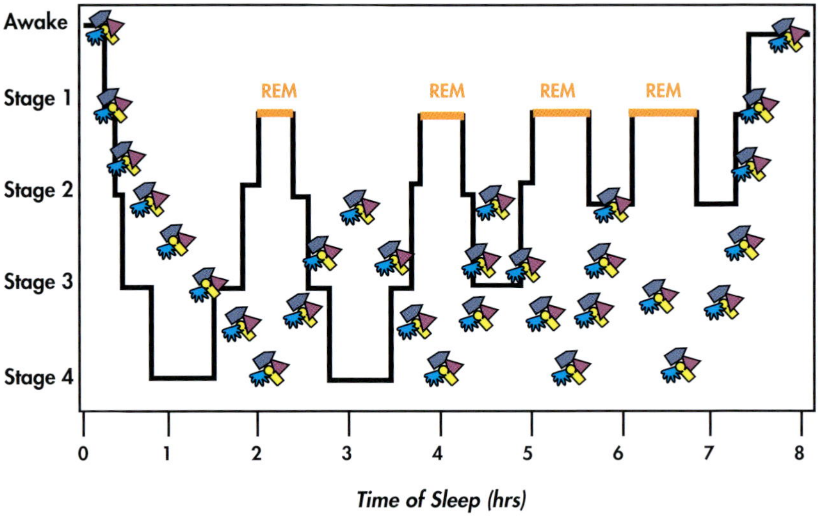

FIGURE 1.21. Dopamine, norepinephrine, serotonin, and histamine levels demonstrate a different trend. They peak during stage 2 sleep and are at their lowest during REM sleep.

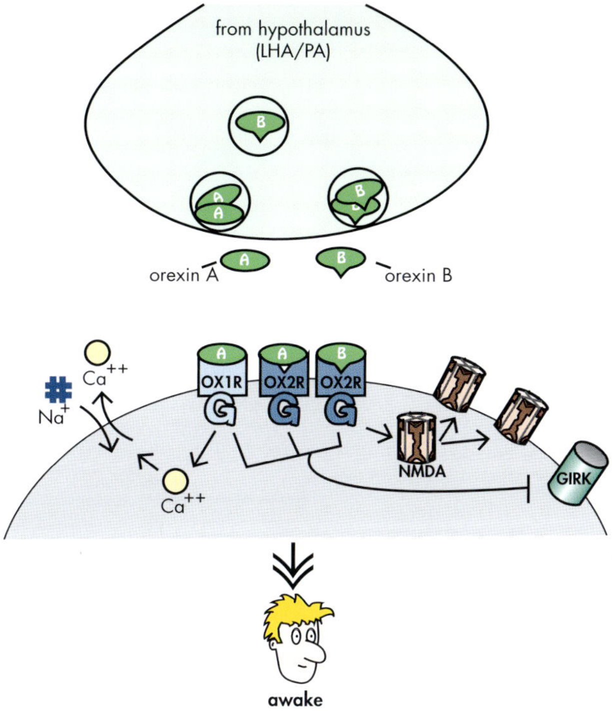

FIGURE 1.22. Hypocretin/orexin neurotransmission is mediated by 2 types of postsynaptic G-protein-coupled receptors, orexin 1 (Ox1R) and orexin 2 (Ox2R). The neurotransmitter orexin A is capable of interacting with both Ox1R and Ox2R, whereas the neurotransmitter orexin B binds selectively to Ox2R. The binding of orexin A to Ox1R leads to increased intracellular calcium as well as activation of the sodium/calcium exchanger. The binding of orexin A or B to Ox2R leads to increased expression of N-methyl-D-aspartate (NMDA) glutamate receptors as well as inactivation of G-protein-regulated inwardly rectifying potassium (GIRK) channels. Ox1R are highly expressed in the noradrenergic locus coeruleus, whereas Ox2R are highly expressed in the histaminergic tuberomammillary nucleus (TMN) (Stahl, 2013).

Hypocretin/Orexin and Motivated Behaviors

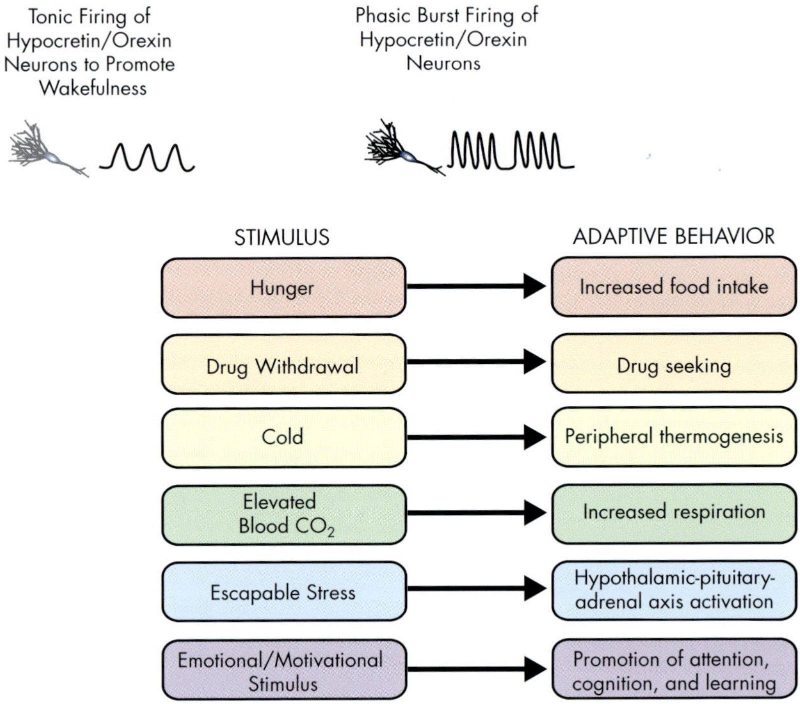

FIGURE 1.23. During periods of wakefulness and partly under the control of the circadian drive from light/dark cycles, hypocretin/orexin neurons are active and fire with tonic frequency to maintain arousal. When presented with a stimulus (either external, such as an escapable stressor, or internal, such as elevated CO_2 levels), hypocretin/orexin neurons exhibit a more rapid phasic burst firing pattern. This excitement of hypocretin/orexin neurons leads to increased neurotransmission and the activation of other brain areas and peripheral responses, which in turn leads to the execution of appropriate behavioral responses. These behavioral responses lead to the attainment of reward or the avoidance of potential danger. In this way, the hypocretin/orexin system not only mediates wakefulness, but also allows for the facilitation of goal-directed, motivated behaviors, including increased food intake in response to hunger (Mahler et al., 2014).

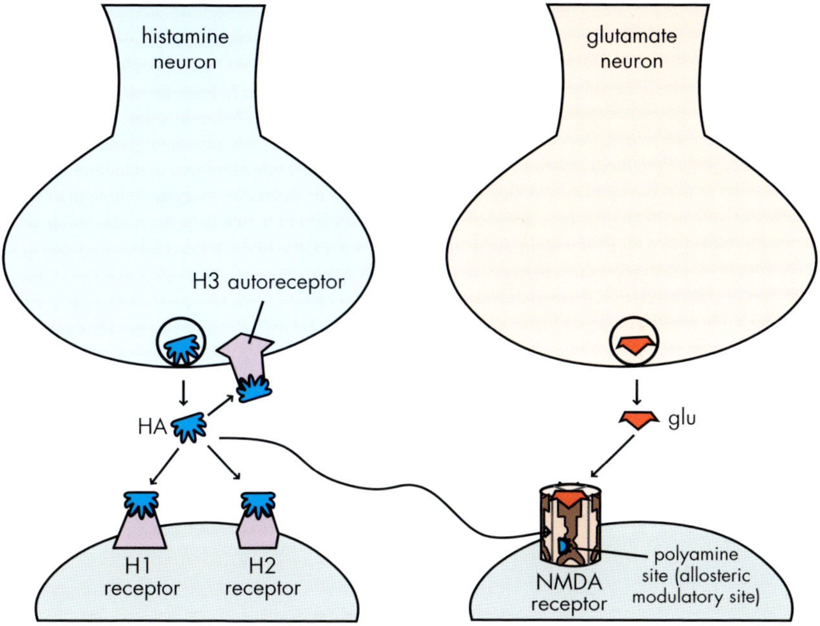

FIGURE 1.24. Shown here are receptors for histamine that regulate its neurotransmission. Histamine 1 and histamine 2 receptors are postsynaptic, while histamine 3 receptors are presynaptic autoreceptors. There is also a binding site for histamine on NMDA receptors; it can act at the polyamine site, which is an allosteric modulatory site (Stahl, 2013).

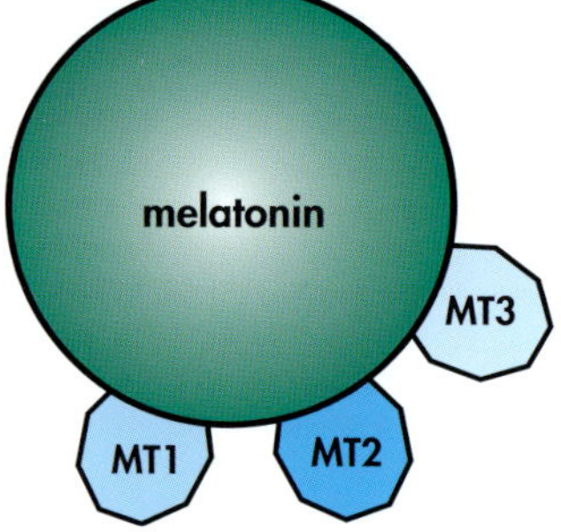

FIGURE 1.25. Endogenous melatonin is secreted by the pineal gland and mainly acts in the suprachiasmatic nucleus to regulate circadian rhythms (see figure 1.7). There are 3 types of receptors for melatonin: melatonin 1 and 2 (MT1 and MT2), which are both involved in sleep, and melatonin 3 (MT3), which is not thought to be involved in sleep physiology (Stahl, 2013).

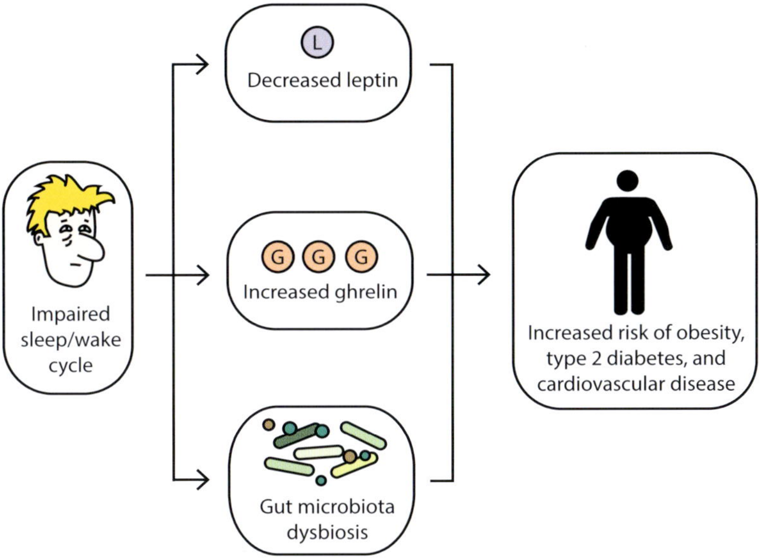

FIGURE 1.26. In recent years, much interest in the relationship between sleep and cardiometabolic issues such as type 2 diabetes and obesity has been expressed. Although much remains unknown, an impaired sleep/wake cycle has been shown to disrupt the circulating levels of both the anorectic (appetite-inhibiting) hormone leptin and the orexigenic (appetite-stimulating) hormone ghrelin. These changes lead to dysfunctional insulin, glucose, and lipid metabolism, which in turn may increase the risk of obesity, type 2 diabetes, and cardiovascular disease (Froy, 2010; Orzel-Gryglewska, 2010; Golombek et al., 2013). Additionally, an altered sleep/wake cycle has been shown to disturb the natural fluctuations in gut microbiota, perhaps further promoting glucose intolerance and obesity (Thaiss et al., 2014).

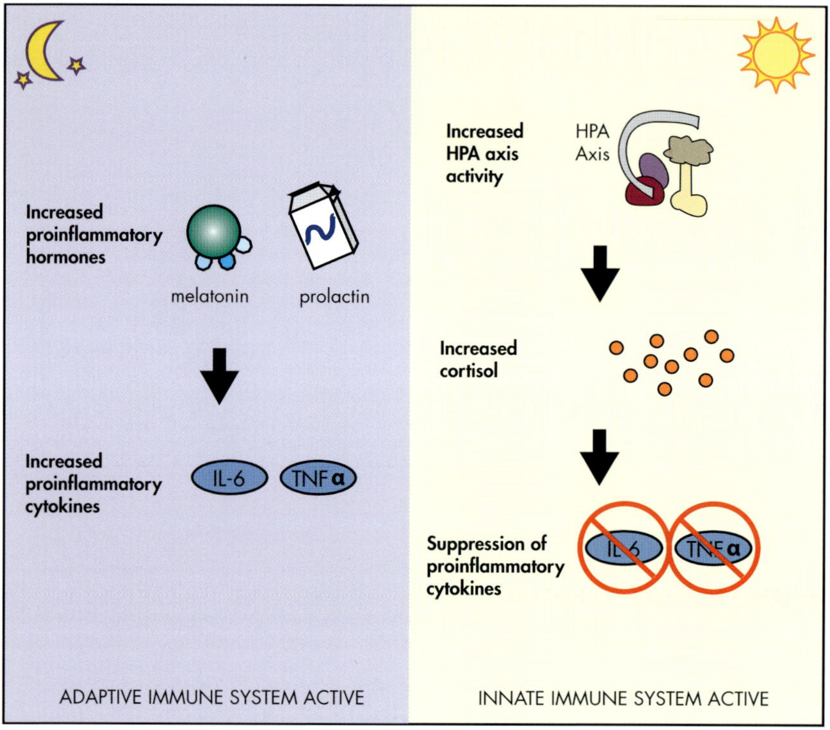

FIGURE 1.27. There are many associations between the sleep/wake cycle and immunity. During the night, there is an increased release of proinflammatory hormones such as prolactin and melatonin, an increased release of proinflammatory cytokines such as IL-6 and TNF alpha, and increased activity in cells of the adaptive (antigen-specific) immune system (i.e., B- and T-lymphocytes). In contrast, daytime brings about increased activity of the hypothalamic-pituitary-adrenal (HPA) axis, increased cortisol release, the suppression of proinflammatory cytokines and allergic reactions, and increased activity of the innate (non-antigen-specific) immune system (i.e., granulocytes, monocytes, and natural killer (NK) cells) (Cermakian et al., 2013). When the sleep/wake cycle is disrupted, this circadian function of the immune system is altered and may lead to immunodeficiency (and, consequently, decreased tumor surveillance) as well as systemic inflammation (Dresler et al., 2104; Golombek et al., 2013).

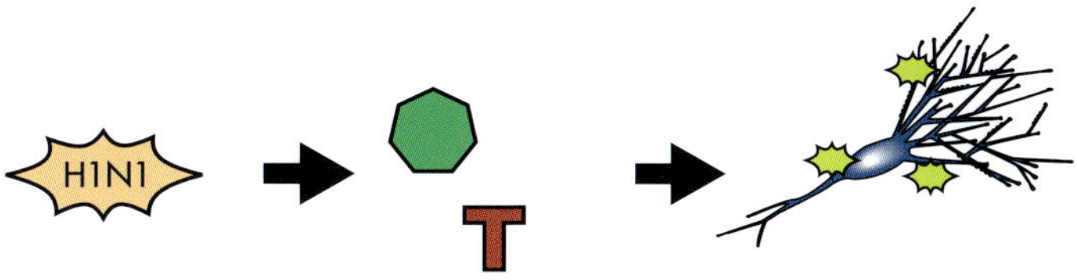

FIGURE 1.28. Both genetic and epidemiological data indicate that the profound loss of hypocretin/orexin (Hcrt/Ox) neurons seen in narcolepsy with cataplexy may be caused by an autoimmune reaction. An increase in the risk of developing narcolepsy has been seen following infection with the H1N1 influenza as well as the H1N1 vaccine (De la Herran-Arita and Garcia-Garcia, 2014). Additionally, genetic studies have shown a strong relationship between narcolepsy and polymorphisms in 2 key components of the immune system: the human leukocyte antigen (HLA) DBQ1-0602 gene and the T-cell receptor alpha gene (Sehgal and Mignot, 2011). It is therefore hypothesized that environmental exposure to certain antigens that are processed by HLA proteins (e.g., H1N1 influenza epitopes), lead to the activation of T cells and may cause an autoimmune reaction that results in the destruction of Hcrt/Ox neurons in genetically predisposed individuals.

2

Assessment of Hypersomnia

There are numerous, often co-occurring, causes of hypersomnia. Optimizing patient outcomes relies on accurately identifying the reasons for hypersomnia and addressing the underlying neurobiological and behavioral causes when possible. Chapter 2 discusses the diagnostic tools available for assessing the degree of hypersomnia as well as strategies for determining the etiology of hypersomnia so that appropriate treatments can be initiated.

Tools for Assessing Sleep/Wake Disorders: Polysomnography

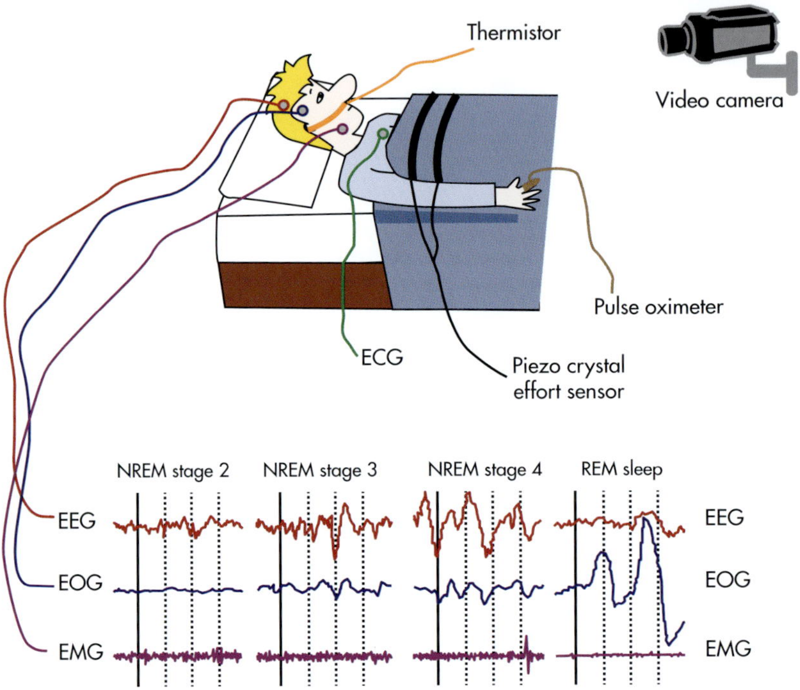

FIGURE 2.1. During polysomnography, an electroencephalogram (EEG) determines sleep stages; an electrooculogram (EOG) measures eye movement to identify rapid eye movement (REM) sleep; and an electromyogram (EMG) measures muscle movement via electrodes on the chin, jaw bone, and calf muscles. In addition, an electrocardiogram (ECG) is used to measure heart rate and rhythm, and breathing is measured with a piezo crystal effort sensor, which utilizes 2 Velcro bands around the chest and abdomen to measure movements and effort. Airflow is measured with a thermistor secured under the nose, and oxygen saturation can be measured by a pulse oximeter on the finger or ear lobe. Finally, the patient may be videotaped (Stahl, 2013).

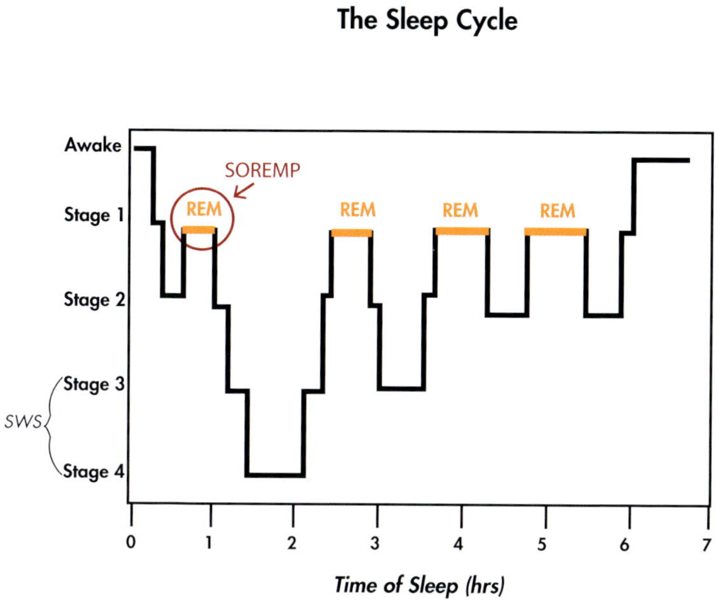

FIGURE 2.2. In healthy individuals, rapid eye movement (REM) sleep occurs approximately 90-110 minutes after sleep onset. However, in individuals with narcolepsy, sleep onset REM periods (SOREMPs) often occur. These abnormal periods of REM sleep occur within 20 minutes of sleep onset. The presence of 2 or more SOREMPs along with a short sleep onset latency (<8 minutes) is diagnostic of narcolepsy (Ahmed and Thorpy, 2010; Adenuga and Attarian, 2014).

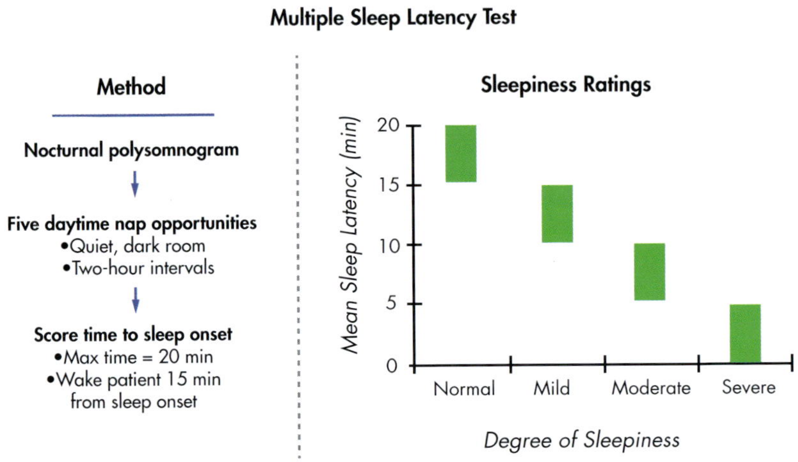

FIGURE 2.3. The Multiple Sleep Latency Test (MSLT) is the most commonly used method for diagnosing sleep disorders. The test requires polysomnography equipment and must be performed by trained physicians in an accredited sleep lab. The degree of sleepiness is measured as the latency to the onset of any stage of sleep, with a mean latency of fewer than 10 minutes usually indicating excessive sleepiness related to a sleep disorder. The Maintenance of Wakefulness Test is a similar test in which the patient is instructed to try to stay awake rather than try to fall asleep, as in the MSLT. Because there are different mechanisms for arousal maintenance and sleep induction, these tests can measure different aspects of excessive sleepiness. Association between scores on these 2 measures is not uniform across disorders; thus, sleep studies should involve both measures (Sangal et al., 1992).

Tools for Assessing Sleep/Wake Disorders: Actigraphy

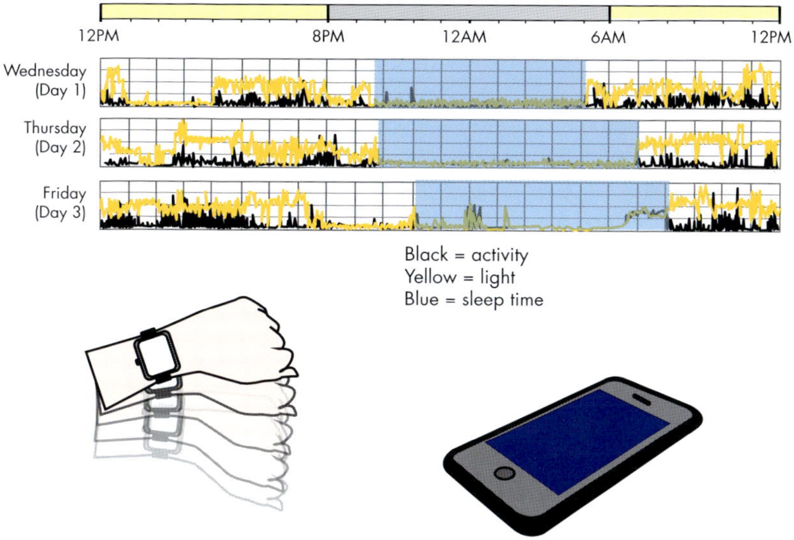

FIGURE 2.4. Actigraphy is used to record body movement over time in order to help assess sleep/wake patterns, including total sleep time and wake after sleep onset (WASO). Actigraphs are available as lightweight devices that can be worn on the wrist and not only record movement, but also sense light (Martin and Hakim, 2011). In fact, there are now several smartphone apps available that can assess not only movement, but also noises, including snoring. At this time, these apps are not quite as accurate as laboratory measures but offer useful tools for in-home monitoring of sleep/wake issues and treatment effectiveness (Stippig et al., 2015).

Tools for Assessing Sleep/Wake Disorders: Sleep/Wake Diary

	Name							
Complete in the Morning	Today's date (include month/day/year):	Mon*	Tues	Wed	Thurs	Fri	Sat	Sun
	Time I went to bed last night: Time I woke up this morning: No. of hours slept last night:	11 p.m. 7 a.m. 8						
	Number of awakenings and total time awake last night:	5 times 2 hrs						
	How long I took to fall asleep last night:	30 mins.						
	How awake did I feel when I got up this morning? 1—Wide awake 2—Awake but a little tired 3—Sleepy	2						
Complete in the Evening	Number of caffeinated drinks (coffee, tea, cola) and time when I had them today:	1 drink at 8 p.m.						
	Number of alcoholic drinks (beer, wine, liquor) and time when I had them today:	2 drinks 9 p.m.						
	Nap times and lengths today:	3:30 p.m. 45 mins.						
	Exercise times and lengths today:	None						
	How sleepy did I feel during the day today? 1—So sleepy had to struggle to stay awake druing much of the day 2—Somewhat tired 3—Fairly alert 4—Wide awake	1						
	*This column shows example diary entries—use as a model for your own diary notes							

FIGURE 2.5. Having patients keep a sleep/wake diary for 1–2 weeks can be very useful in assessing the contribution of poor sleep hygiene or medication use to sleep/wake problems.

Tools for Assessing Sleep/Wake Disorders: Epworth Sleepiness Scale

The Epworth Sleepiness Scale

How likely are you to dose off or fall asleep in the following situations, in contrast to just feeling tired? This refers to your usual way of life in recent times. Even if you have not done some of these things recently, try to work out how they would have affected you. Use the following scale to choose the most appropraite number for each situation:

0=Would never doze	2=Moderate chance of dozing
1=Slight chance of dozing	3=High chance of dozing

Situation	**Chance of Dozing**
Sitting and reading	________
Watching TV	________
Sitting inactive in a public place (e.g., a theater or a meeting)	________
As a passenger in a car for an hour without a break	________
Lying down to rest in the afternoon when circumstance permit	________
Sitting and talking to someone	________
Sitting quietly after a lunch without alcohol	________
In a car, while stopped for a few minutes in traffic	________

FIGURE 2.6. The Epworth Sleepiness Scale (ESS) is a self-rated, subjective measure of sleepiness. It is useful as a point-of-care tool for rapidly assessing the severity of sleepiness in a patient. For the general population, the average score on the ESS is approximately 5.9; a score over 11 indicates excessive sleepiness (Stahl, 2013).

Tools for Assessing Sleep/Wake Disorders: Pittsburgh Sleep Quality Index

During the past month, how often have you had trouble sleeping because you:				
	Not during the past month	Less than once a week	1-2 times a week	3+ times a week
a) Cannot get to sleep within 30 minutes				
b) Wake up in the middle of the night or early morning				
c) Have to get up to use the bathroom				
d) Cannot breathe comfortbaly				
e) Cough or snore loudly				
f) Feel too cold				
g) Feel too hot				
h) Had bad dreams				
i) Have pain				

FIGURE 2.7. The Pittsburgh Sleep Quality Index (PSQI) provides a self-reported measure of sleep quality and is useful for assessing insomnia (Buysse et al., 1989). The full PSQI as well as the scoring algorithm can be found at http://www.sleep.pitt.edu.

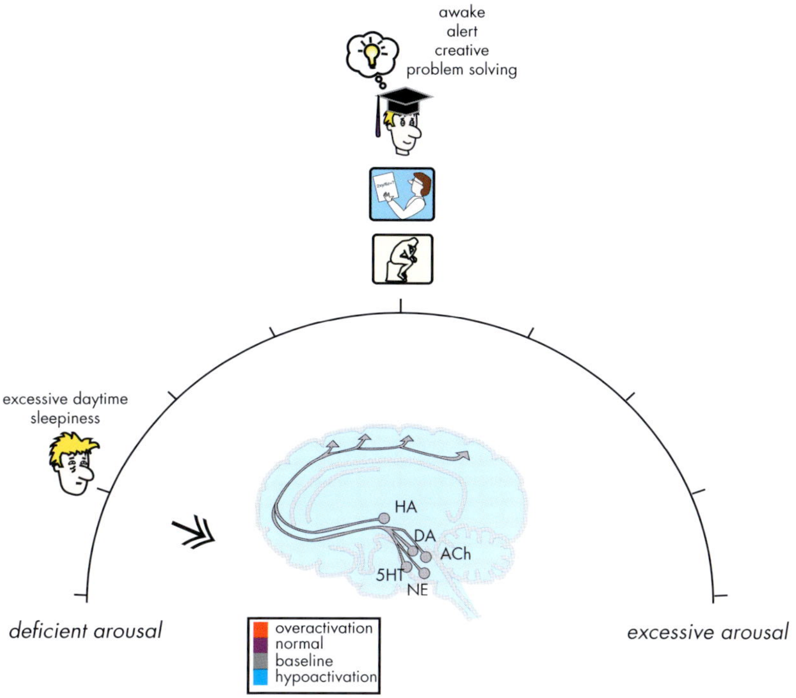

FIGURE 2.8. Excessive sleepiness is conceptualized as being related to hypoarousal during the day, depicted here as the brain being blue (hypoactive) (Stahl, 2013).

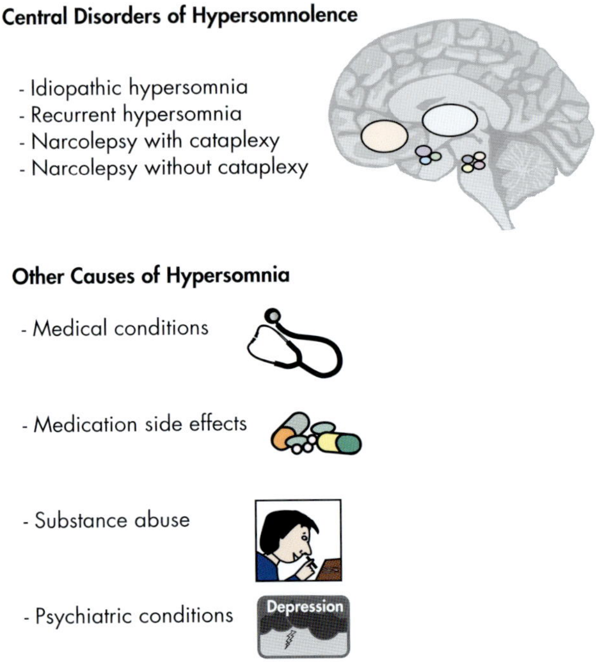

FIGURE 2.9. Hypersomnia is present in as much as 6% of the population (Dresler et al., 2014). Hypersomnia can occur in association with other sleep/wake disorders, medical conditions, medication side effects, or psychiatric illnesses (Adenuga and Attarian, 2014). In fact, as many as 25% of individuals with hypersomnia may have a mood disorder (Larson-Prior et al., 2014; Morgenthaler et al., 2007). There are also several disorders of hypersomnia that are not secondary to these other conditions and are thought to arise as a consequence of neuropathology in the sleep/wake circuitry of the brain. Such disorders are known as "central disorders of hypersomnolence" and include idiopathic hypersomnia, recurrent hypersomnia, and narcolepsy. With the exception of narcolepsy with cataplexy, the underlying neuropathology of the central disorders of hypersomnolence is largely unknown.

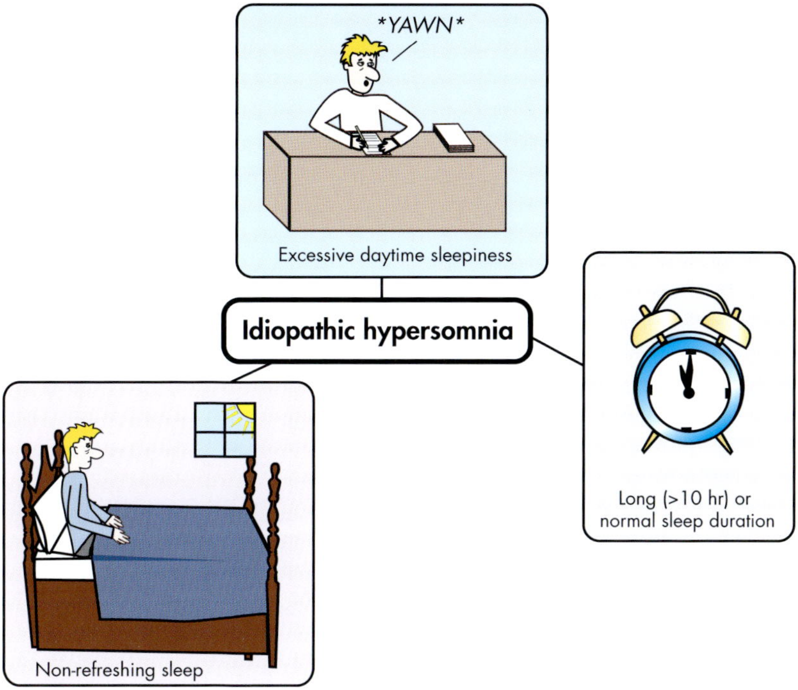

FIGURE 2.10. Idiopathic hypersomnia is characterized by either long or normal sleep duration accompanied by constant excessive daytime sleepiness, short sleep onset latency, and complaints of non-refreshing sleep. Patients with idiopathic hypersomnia may also report sleep drunkenness and somnolence following sleep. The diagnosis of idiopathic hypersomnia includes excessive daytime sleepiness lasting at least 3 months; a sleep latency of under 8 minutes, as determined by the Multiple Sleep Latency Test (MSLT); and fewer than 2 sleep onset REM periods (SOREMPs). Cerebrospinal fluid (CSF) levels of histamine may be low; however, unlike in narcolepsy with cataplexy, hypocretin levels are not typically affected (Dresler et al., 2014). Polysomnography should be performed to rule out other causes of hypersomnolence, and psychiatric and medical evaluations are also warranted, as idiopathic hypersomnia is often accompanied by memory and attention deficits, digestive system problems, depression, and anxiety (Larson-Prior et al., 2014; Morgenthaler et al., 2007).

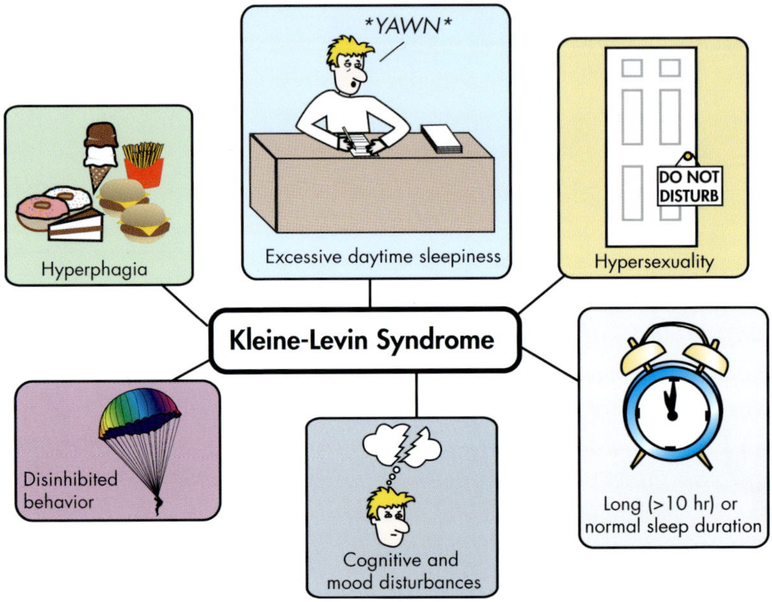

FIGURE 2.11. Recurrent hypersomnia is characterized by continuing excessive daytime sleepiness and may be associated with menstruation in women. However, Kleine-Levin syndrome is the most common form of recurrent hypersomnia. This rare disorder mostly affects adolescent boys and is characterized by bouts of hypersomnolence coupled with cognitive and mood disturbances, compulsive eating, hypersexuality, and disinhibited behavior (Dresler et al., 2014; Larson-Prior et al., 2014). Interestingly, accumulating data suggest an etiology of viral infection and subsequent autoimmune reaction, making Kleine-Levin syndrome similar to narcolepsy in that aspect (Larson-Prior et al., 2014; Morgenthaler et al., 2007).

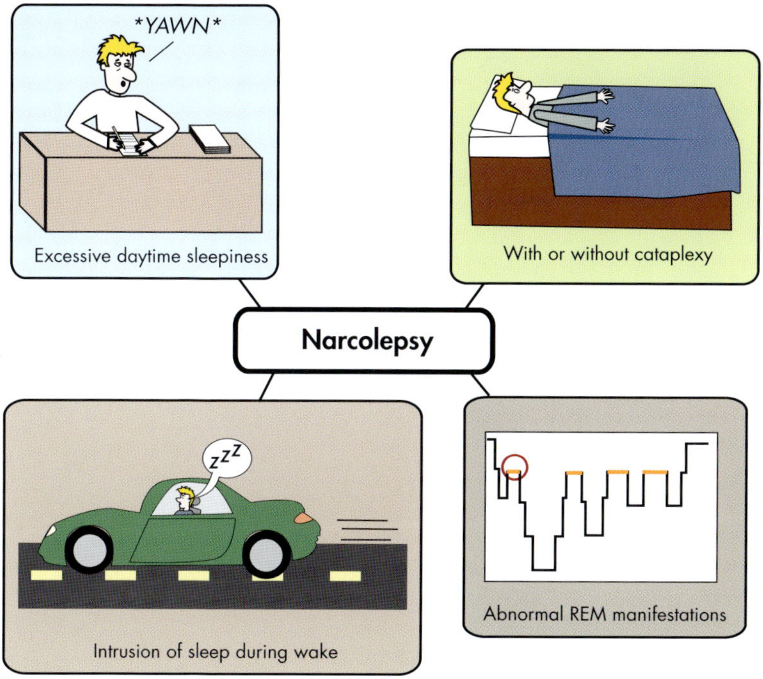

FIGURE 2.12. Narcolepsy is characterized by excessive daytime sleepiness, intrusion of sleep during periods of wakefulness, and abnormal REM sleep, including periods of REM occurring at the onset of sleep (SOREMPs). Cataplexy, or loss of muscle tone triggered by emotions, may also be present. Hypnagogic hallucinations, which are present upon waking, are also often present (Adenuga and Attarian, 2014).

The Neurobiology of Narcolepsy With Cataplexy

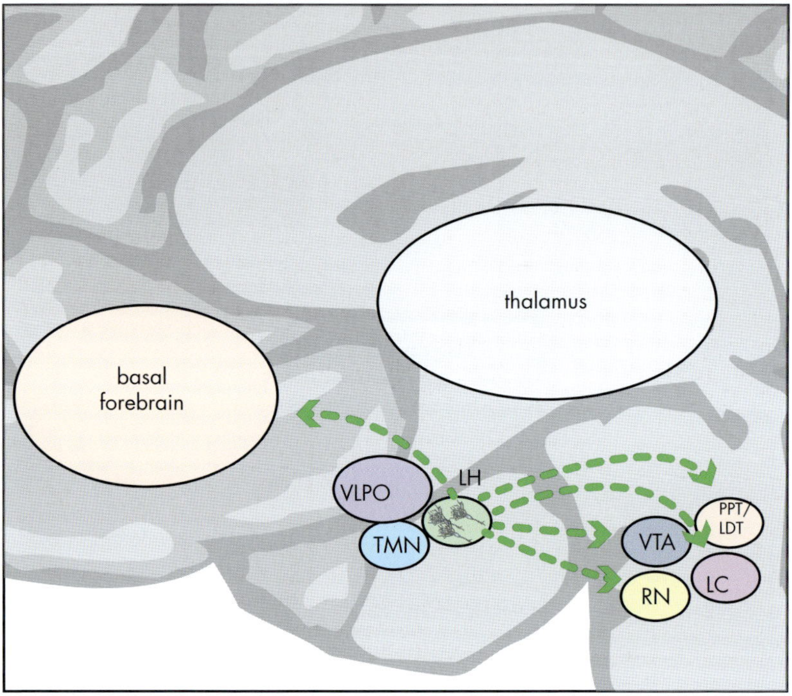

FIGURE 2.13. A clear neuropathological substrate has been identified for narcolepsy with cataplexy. Patients with narcolepsy with cataplexy exhibit a profound loss of hypocretin/orexin neurons in the lateral hypothalamus. These neurons are involved in the maintenance of wakefulness through their actions on other components of the wake circuit. Additionally, the input of hypocretin/orexin neurons stimulates norepinephrine from the locus coeruleus and serotonin from the raphe nucleus. The release of norepinephrine and serotonin influences the activation of motor neurons. During REM sleep, norepinephrine and serotonin activation of motor activity as well as components of the wake circuit are inhibited via GABA released from the ventrolateral preoptic nucleus. Hypocretin/orexin normally prevents this inhibition of motor control during periods of wakefulness by turning off the ventrolateral preoptic nucleus. Given that hypocretin/orexin is necessary for the stabilization of wakefulness, it is not surprising that patients with loss of hypocretin/orexin neurons exhibit intrusion of sleep and cataplexy during periods of wakefulness (Adenuga and Attarian, 2014).

The Differential Diagnosis of Hypersomnia

	Subjective Sleepiness	MSLT Sleep Latency	SOREMPs	Hcrt/Ox Levels
Narcolepsy with cataplexy	✓	≤ 8 min	≥ 2	Low ≤110 pg/mL
Narcolepsy without cataplexy	✓	≤ 8 min	≥ 2	Normal 200-700 pg/mL
Idiopathic hypersomnia	✓	≤ 8 min	< 2	Normal 200-700 pg/mL
Recurrent hypersomnia	✓ Episodic	Normal between episodes	< 2	Normal 200-700 pg/mL

FIGURE 2.14. It is important to first eliminate and treat secondary causes of hypersomnia, such as obstructive sleep apnea, psychiatric illnesses, and medication side effects. This can be accomplished by conducting a full clinical interview, collecting data from a sleep/wake diary and 1–2 weeks' worth of actigraphy, and performing polysomnography (PSG) as well as the Multiple Sleep Latency Test (MSLT) (Ahmed and Thorpy, 2010). A cerebrospinal fluid (CSF) hypocretin/orexin (Hcrt/Ox) level of <110 pg/mL is diagnostic for narcolepsy; however, Hcrt/Ox levels are often within normal range in narcolepsy, especially without cataplexy, as well as idiopathic and recurrent hypersomnia (Bourgin et al., 2008). Even in the absence of low Hcrt/Ox levels, patients with narcolepsy with or without cataplexy demonstrate ≥2 SOREMPs on the MSLT or 1 SOREMP on PSG as well as a short sleep latency (≤8 minutes) on the MSLT; thus, these measures are also considered diagnostic for narcolepsy (Dresler et al., 2014). Additionally, the majority (90%) of patients with narcolepsy, particularly those with cataplexy, are positive for the HLA DQB1-0602 polymorphism compared to only 20% in the general population (Mignot, 2012).

3 Treatment of Hypersomnia

Chapter 3 discusses pharmacological and nonpharmacological strategies for the treatment of disorders of hypersomnolence. These treatments are often aimed at reestablishing healthy circadian rhythms, reducing excessive daytime sleepiness, and in the case of narcolepsy, reducing cataplexy. Prescribing tips and pearls for many of these agents are discussed; however, clinicians should consult the full prescribing information provided by the manufacturer before initiating any pharmacological agent. This chapter also includes discussion of novel agents that are currently undergoing trials and may be available in the near future.

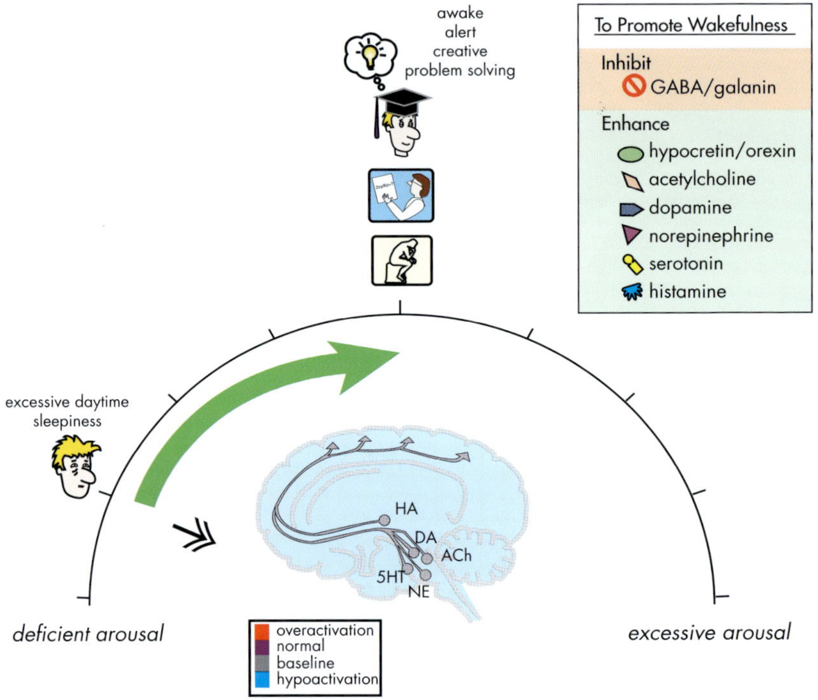

FIGURE 3.1. Agents that increase brain activation, such as the stimulants modafinil and caffeine, can shift one's arousal state from hypoactive to awake with normal alertness (Stahl, 2013). The currently available agents as well as those in development for the treatment of excessive sleepiness target the neurotransmitter systems involved in the sleep and wake circuits, inhibiting the neurotransmitters that promote sleep and/or enhancing the systems that promote wakefulness.

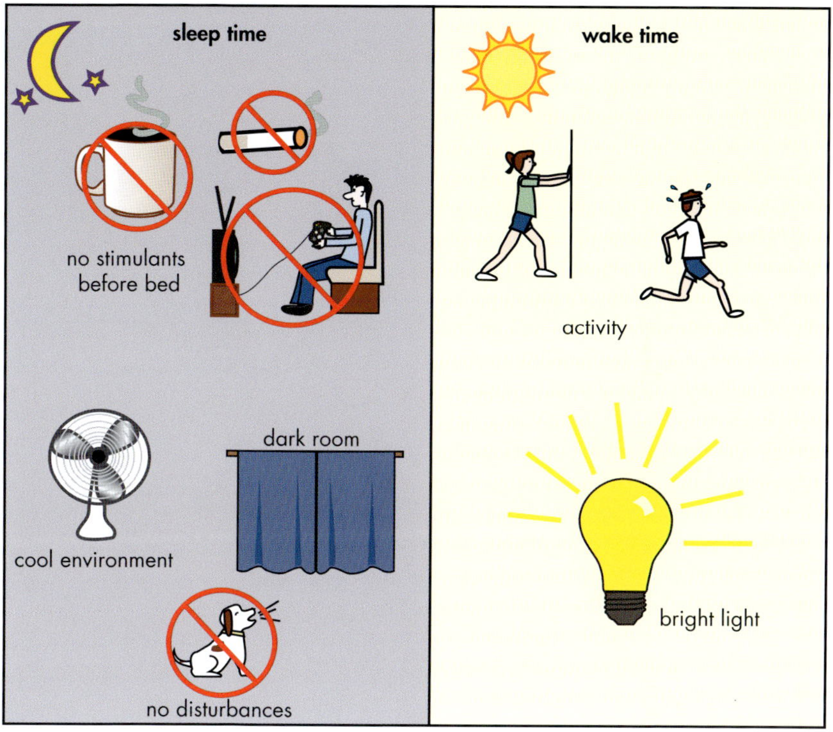

FIGURE 3.2. Good sleep hygiene involves using the bed exclusively for sleep as opposed to activities such as reading or watching television; avoiding stimulants such as alcohol, caffeine, and nicotine as well as strenuous exercise before bed; limiting time spent awake in bed (if not asleep within 20 minutes, one should get up and return to bed when sleepy); not watching the clock; adopting regular sleep habits; and avoiding bright light at night (Stahl, 2013). In the case of narcolepsy, scheduled naps of 15–20 minutes may also be beneficial (Harris et al., 2012).

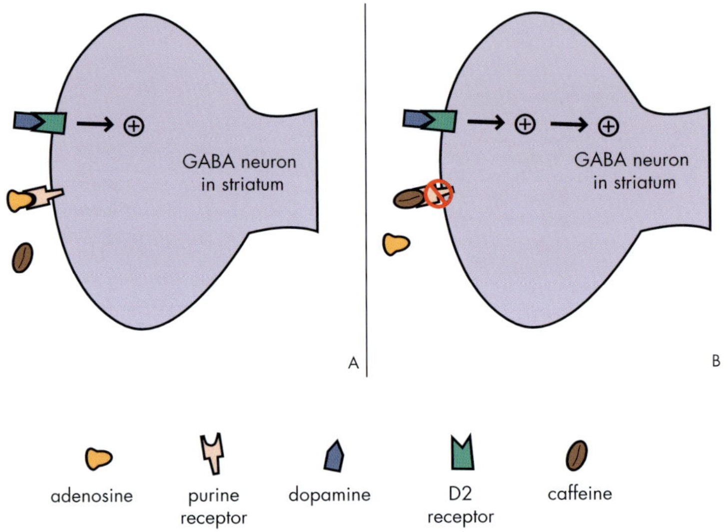

FIGURE 3.3. A) Both adenosine 2A receptors and dopamine D2 receptors are localized on GABAergic neurons in the striatum, forming a heteromeric complex. When adenosine stimulates adenosine 2A receptors, this reduces the affinity of nearby D2 receptors for dopamine. B) By blocking adenosine from binding to adenosine 2A receptors, caffeine prevents the lowered affinity of D2 receptors for dopamine. The increased GABAergic neurotransmission disinhibits downstream excitatory glutamatergic neurotransmission (Morrissette, 2013).

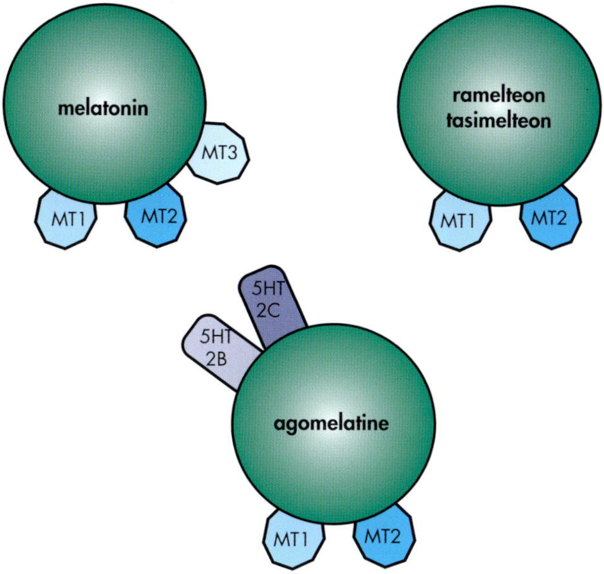

FIGURE 3.4. There are several different agents that act at melatonin receptors, as shown here. Melatonin itself, available over the counter, acts at MT1 and MT2 receptors as well as at the melatonin 3 (MT3) site. Both ramelteon and tasimelteon are MT1 and MT2 receptor agonists and seem to improve sleep onset, though not necessarily sleep maintenance. Agomelatine is not only an MT1 and MT2 receptor agonist, but also a 5HT2C and 5HT2B receptor antagonist; it is available as an antidepressant in Europe (Stahl, 2013). Although used in the treatment of insomnia, these melatonergic agents may also be useful in the treatment of disorders of hypersomnolence because they reset circadian rhythms that may be out of tune (Stahl, 2013).

The Pharmacological Treatment of Hypersomnia

	Excessive Daytime Sleepiness	Cataplexy
Stimulants		
Amphetamine	*✓	
Methylphenidate	*✓	
Lisdexamfetamine	✓	
Atomoxetine	✓	✓
Antidepressants		
TCA -Protriptyline		✓
TCA -Imipramine		✓
TCA -Clomipramine		✓
TCA -Desipramine		✓
SNRI -Venlafaxine		✓
SNRI -Duloxetine		✓
SSRI -Fluoxetine		✓
MAOI -Selegiline	✓	✓
Other Agents		
Modafinil/Armodafinil	*✓	
Sodium Oxybate	*✓	*✓

* Indicates FDA approval for this indication

FIGURE 3.5. Pharmacological agents used in the treatment of excessive daytime sleepiness and cataplexy include stimulants and antidepressants as well as sodium oxybate and the wake-promoting agent modafinil/armodafinil (Hirai and Nishino, 2011; Mignot, 2012; Thorpy and Dauvilliers, 2014; Zaharna et al., 2010). In many cases, a combination of agents may be required to optimize symptom control in patients with hypersomnia.

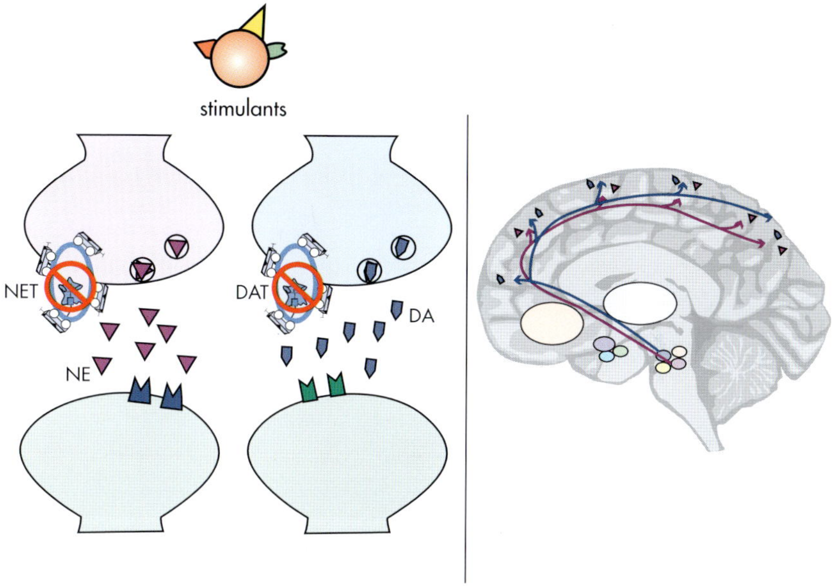

FIGURE 3.6. Stimulants, including amphetamine and methylphenidate, act in part by inhibiting dopamine (DA) and/or norepinephrine reuptake transporters (DAT and NET, respectively), thus increasing the levels of dopamine (DA) and norepinephrine (NE) in the wake circuit. Atomoxetine has a similar mechanism of action involving the inhibition of norepinephrine reuptake (Hirai and Nishino, 2011; Mignot, 2012).

Prescribing Tips: Amphetamine (D)

Commonly Prescribed for *(bold for FDA-approved)*

- **ADHD (ages 6 and older; ages 3–5 for Dextro Stat)**
- **Narcolepsy**
- Treatment-resistant depression

Usual Dosage Range

- 5–60 mg/day (divided doses for tablet, once daily morning dose for Spansule capsule)

Dosage Forms

- Spansule capsule: 5 mg, 10 mg, 15 mg
- Tablet: 5 mg scored, 10 mg

How to Dose

- Initial dose 10 mg/day; increase by 10 mg each week; give first dose on waking
- Can give once daily dosing with Spansule capsule or divided dosing with tablet (every 4–6 hours)

Habit Forming

- High abuse potential, Schedule II drug

Side Effects

- Insomnia, headache, exacerbation of tics, nervousness, irritability, overstimulation, tremor, dizziness
- Anorexia, nausea, dry mouth, constipation, diarrhea, weight loss
- Can temporarily slow normal growth in children (controversial)

Life-threatening or Dangerous Side Effects

- Psychotic episodes, especially with parenteral abuse
- Seizures
- Palpitations, tachycardia, hypertension
- Rare activation of hypomania, mania, or suicidal ideation (controversial)
- Cardiovascular adverse effects, sudden death in patients with preexisting cardiac structural abnormalities

Potential Advantages

- Established long-term efficacy of immediate-release and Spansule formulations

Potential Disadvantages

- Patients with current or past substance abuse
- Patients with current or past bipolar disorder or psychosis

FIGURE 3.7. Prescribing information for amphetamine (D) (Stahl, 2014).

Prescribing Tips: Amphetamine (D,L)

Commonly Prescribed for *(bold for FDA-approved)*
- **ADHD in children ages 3–12 (Adderall)**
- **ADHD in children ages 6–17 and adults (Adderall XR)**
- **Narcolepsy (Adderall)**
- Treatment-resistant depression

Usual Dosage Range
- 5–60 mg/day in divided doses

Dosage Forms
- Immediate-release tablet: 5 mg double scored, 7.5 mg double scored, 10 mg double scored, 12.5 mg double scored, 15 mg double scored, 20 mg double scored, 30 mg double scored
- Extended-release tablet: 5 mg, 10 mg, 15 mg, 20 mg, 25 mg, 30 mg

How to Dose
- Immediate-release formulation in narcolepsy (ages 12 and older): initial dose 10 mg/day; increase by 10 mg each week; give first dose on waking and every 4–6 hours thereafter
- Extended-release formulation in ADHD: initial dose 10 mg/day in the morning; can increase by 5–10 mg/day at weekly intervals; maximum dose generally 30 mg/day

Habit Forming
- High abuse potential, Schedule II drug
- Patients may develop tolerance, psychological dependence

Side Effects
- Insomnia, headache, exacerbation of tics, nervousness, irritability, overstimulation, tremor, dizziness
- Anorexia, nausea, dry mouth, constipation, diarrhea, weight loss
- Can temporarily slow normal growth in children (controversial)

Life-threatening or Dangerous Side Effects
- Psychotic episodes, especially with parenteral abuse
- Seizures
- Palpitations, tachycardia, hypertension
- Rare activation of hypomania, mania, or suicidal ideation (controversial)
- Cardiovascular adverse effects, sudden death in patients with preexisting cardiac structural abnormalities

Potential Advantages
- New sustained-release option

Potential Disadvantages
- Patients with current or past substance abuse
- Patients with current or past bipolar disorder or psychosis

FIGURE 3.8. Prescribing information for amphetamine (D,L) (Stahl, 2014).

Prescribing Tips: Methylphenidate (D)

Commonly Prescribed for *(bold for FDA-approved)*

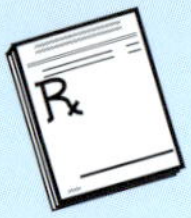

- **ADHD in children ages 6–17 (Focalin, Focalin XR) and adults (Focalin XR)**
- Narcolepsy
- Treatment-resistant depression

Usual Dosage Range

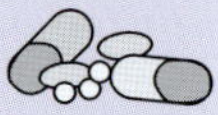

- 2.5–10 mg twice per day

Dosage Forms
- Tablet: 2.5 mg, 5 mg, 10 mg
- Extended-release capsule: 5 mg, 10 mg, 15 mg, 20 mg, 25 mg, 30 mg, 35 mg, 40 mg

How to Dose
- Immediate-release: for patients not taking racemic d,l-methylphenidate, initial dose 2.5 mg twice per day in 4-hour intervals; may adjust dose in weekly intervals by 2.5–5 mg/day; maximum dose generally 10 mg twice per day
- Immediate-release: for patients currently taking racemic d,l-methylphenidate, initial dose should be half the current dose of racemic d,l-methylphenidate; maximum dose generally 10 mg twice per day
- Extended-release: for children, same titration schedule as immediate-release but dosed once in the morning; maximum dose 30 mg/day
- Extended-release: for adults not taking racemic d,l-methylphenidate, initial dose 10 mg/day in the morning; may adjust dose in weekly intervals by 10 mg/day; maximum dose generally 40 mg/day

Habit Forming
- High abuse potential, Schedule II drug
- Patients may develop tolerance, psychological dependence

Side Effects

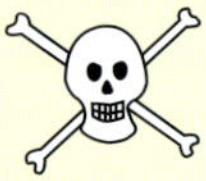

- Insomnia, headache, exacerbation of tics, nervousness, irritability, overstimulation, tremor, dizziness
- Anorexia, nausea, abdominal pain, weight loss
- Can temporarily slow normal growth in children (controversial)
- Blurred vision

Life-threatening or Dangerous Side Effects
- Psychotic episodes, especially with parenteral abuse
- Rare priapism
- Seizures
- Palpitations, tachycardia, hypertension
- Rare neuroleptic malignant syndrome
- Rare activation of hypomania, mania, or suicidal ideation (controversial)
- Cardiovascular adverse effects, sudden death in patients with preexisting cardiac structural abnormalities

Potential Advantages

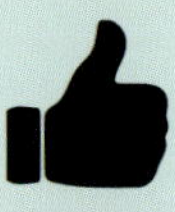

- Established long-term efficacy as a first-line treatment for ADHD
- Multiple options for drug delivery, peak actions, and duration of action

Potential Disadvantages

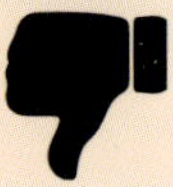

- Patients with current or past substance abuse
- Patients with current or past bipolar disorder or psychosis

FIGURE 3.9. Prescribing information for methylphenidate (D) (Stahl, 2014).

Prescribing Tips: Methylphenidate (D,L)

Commonly Prescribed for *(bold for FDA-approved)*
- **ADHD in children and adults (approved ages vary based on formulation)**
- **Narcolepsy (Metadate ER, Methylin ER, Ritalin, Ritalin SR)**
- Treatment-resistant depression

Usual Dosage Range
- 20–60 mg/day in 2–3 divided doses

Dosage Forms
- Immediate-release tablet: 5 mg, 10 mg, 20 mg (Ritalin, Methylin, generic methylphenidate)
- Immediate-release chewable tablet: 2.5 mg, 5 mg, 10 mg
- Oral solution: 5 mg/mL, 10 mg/5 mL
- Older sustained-release tablet: 10 mg, 20 mg (Metadate ER, Methylin ER); 20 mg (Ritalin SR)
- Newer sustained-release capsule: 20 mg, 30 mg, 40 mg (Ritalin LA); 10 mg, 20 mg, 30 mg (Metadate CD)
- Newer sustained-release tablet: 18 mg, 27 mg, 36 mg, 54 mg (Concerta)
- Transdermal patch: 27 mg/12.5 cm2 (10 mg/9 hours), 41.3 mg/18.75 cm2 (15 mg/9 hours), 55 mg/25 cm2 (20 mg/9 hours), 82.5 mg/37.5 cm2 (30 mg/9 hours)

How to Dose
- Varies depending on formulation

Habit Forming
- High abuse potential, Schedule II drug
- Patients may develop tolerance, psychological dependence

Side Effects
- Insomnia, headache, exacerbation of tics, nervousness, irritability, overstimulation, tremor, dizziness
- Anorexia, nausea, abdominal pain, weight loss
- Can temporarily slow normal growth in children (controversial)
- Blurred vision
- Transdermal: application site reactions, including contact sensitization (erythema, edema, papules, vesicles)

Life-threatening or Dangerous Side Effects
- Psychotic episodes, especially with parenteral abuse
- Rare priapism
- Seizures
- Palpitations, tachycardia, hypertension
- Rare neuroleptic malignant syndrome
- Rare activation of hypomania, mania, or suicidal ideation (controversial)
- Cardiovascular adverse effects, sudden death in patients with preexisting cardiac structural abnormalities
- Rare activation of hypomania, mania, or suicidal ideation (controversial)
- Cardiovascular adverse effects, sudden death in patients with preexisting cardiac structural abnormalities

Potential Advantages
- Established long-term efficacy as a first-line treatment for ADHD
- Multiple options for drug delivery, peak actions, and duration of action

Potential Disadvantages
- Patients with current or past substance abuse
- Patients with current or past bipolar disorder or psychosis

FIGURE 3.10. Prescribing information for methylphenidate (D,L) (Stahl, 2014).

Prescribing Tips: Lisdexamfetamine

Commonly Prescribed for *(bold for FDA-approved)*
- **ADHD (ages 6 and older)**
- Narcolepsy
- Treatment-resistant depression

Usual Dosage Range
- 30 mg/day

Dosage Forms
- Capsule: 20 mg, 30 mg, 40 mg, 50 mg, 60 mg, 70 mg

How to Dose
- Initial dose 30 mg/day in the morning; can increase by 10–20 mg each week; maximum dose generally 70 mg/day

Habit Forming
- Schedule II drug
- Patients may develop tolerance, psychological dependence
- Theoretically, less abuse potential than other stimulants when taken as directed because it is inactive until it reaches the gut and thus has delayed time to onset as well as long duration of action

Side Effects
- Insomnia, headache, exacerbation of tics, nervousness, irritability, overstimulation, tremor, dizziness
- Anorexia, nausea, dry mouth, constipation, diarrhea, weight loss
- Can temporarily slow normal growth in children (controversial)

Life-threatening or Dangerous Side Effects
- Psychotic episodes, especially with parenteral abuse
- Seizures
- Palpitations, tachycardia, hypertension
- Rare activation of hypomania, mania, or suicidal ideation (controversial)
- Cardiovascular adverse effects, sudden death in patients with preexisting cardiac structural abnormalities

Potential Advantages
- Although restricted as a Schedule II controlled substance like other stimulants, as a prodrug, lisdexamfetamine may have a lower propensity for abuse, intoxication, or dependence than other stimulants
- May be particularly useful in adult patients without prior diagnosis and treatment of ADHD as a child to prevent abuse and diversion since lisdexamfetamine may be less abusable than other stimulants

Potential Disadvantages
- Patients with current or past substance abuse
- Patients with current or past bipolar disorder or psychosis

FIGURE 3.11. Prescribing information for lisdexamfetamine (Stahl, 2014).

Prescribing Tips: Atomoxetine

Commonly Prescribed for *(bold for FDA-approved)*
- **ADHD in adults and children over 6**
- Treatment-resistant depression

Usual Dosage Range
- 30 mg/day

Dosage Forms
- 0.5–1.2 mg/kg/day in children up to 70 kg; 40–100 mg/day in adults

How to Dose
- For children 70 kg or less: initial dose 0.5 mg/kg per day; after 7 days, can increase to 1.2 mg/kg per day either once in the morning or divided; maximum dose 1.4 mg/kg per day or 100 mg/day, whichever is less
- For children over 70 kg and adults: initial dose 40 mg/day; after 7 days, can increase to 80 mg/day once in the morning or divided; after 2–4 weeks, can increase to 100 mg/day if necessary; maximum daily dose 100 mg

Habit Forming
- No

Side Effects
- Sedation, fatigue (particularly in children)
- Decreased appetite
- Rare priapism
- Increased heart rate (6–9 beats/min)
- Increased blood pressure (2–4 mm Hg)
- Insomnia, dizziness, anxiety, agitation, aggression, irritability
- Dry mouth, constipation, nausea, vomiting, abdominal pain, dyspepsia
- Urinary hesitancy, urinary retention (older men)
- Dysmenorrhea, sweating
- Sexual dysfunction (men: decreased libido, erectile disturbance, impotence, ejaculatory dysfunction, abnormal orgasm; women: decreased libido, abnormal orgasm)

Life-threatening or Dangerous Side Effects
- Increased heart rate and hypertension
- Orthostatic hypotension
- Severe liver damage (rare)
- Hypomania and, theoretically, rare induction of mania
- Rare activation of suicidality

Potential Advantages
- No known abuse potential

Potential Disadvantages
- May not act as rapidly as stimulants when initiating treatment in some patients

FIGURE 3.12. Prescribing information for atomoxetine (Stahl, 2014).

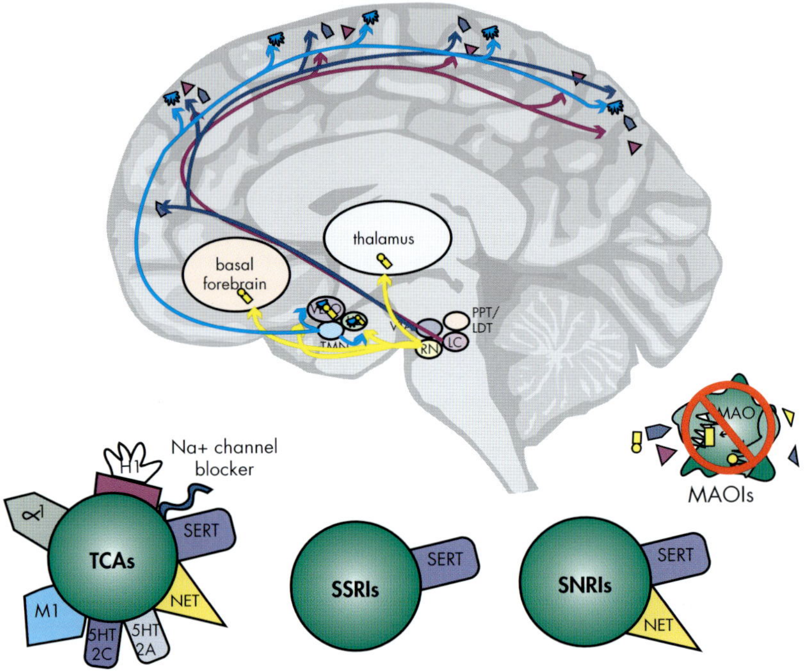

FIGURE 3.13. Antidepressants, including tricyclic antidepressants (TCAs), selective serotonin reuptake inhibitors (SSRIs), and serotonin-norepinephrine reuptake inhibitors (SNRIs) can have beneficial effects on cataplexy by reducing REM sleep. Although monoamine oxidase inhibitors (MAOIs) are perhaps underutilized, there is some evidence to suggest that selegiline may have efficacy in the treatment of both excessive sleepiness and cataplexy (Ahmed and Thorpy, 2010). In addition to its antidepressant actions, selegiline may also be useful in treating cataplexy because it is metabolized into the stimulant amphetamine. However, it is important to note that the cessation of antidepressant treatment may result in rebound cataplexy (Mignot, 2012).

Prescribing Tips: TCAs

Commonly Prescribed for *(bold for FDA-approved)*
- **Depression (imipramine, desipramine)**
- **Mental depression (protriptyline)**
- **Obsessive compulsive disorder (OCD) (clomipramine)**
- Anxiety (imipramine, desipramine, clomipramine)
- Insomnia (imipramine, desipramine, clomipramine)
- Neuropathic pain/chronic pain (imipramine, desipramine, clomipramine)
- Cataplexy syndrome (imipramine, clomipramine)
- Enuresis (imipramine)

Usual Dosage Range
- Imipramine: 50–150 mg/day
- Desipramine: 100–200 mg/day (for depression); 50–150 mg/day (for chronic pain)
- Clomipramine: 100–200 mg/day
- Protriptyline: 15–40 mg/day in 3–4 divided doses

Dosage Forms
- Imipramine: capsule: 75 mg, 100 mg, 125 mg, 150 mg; tablet: 10 mg, 25 mg, 50 mg
- Desipramine: tablet: 10 mg, 25 mg, 50 mg, 75 mg, 100 mg, 150 mg
- Clomipramine: capsule: 25 mg, 50 mg, 75 mg
- Protriptyline: tablet: 5 mg, 10 mg

How to Dose
- Varies depending on agent

Habit Forming
- No

Side Effects
- Blurred vision, constipation, urinary retention, increased appetite, dry mouth, nausea, diarrhea, heartburn, unusual taste in mouth, weight gain
- Fatigue, weakness, dizziness, sedation, headache, anxiety, nervousness, restlessness
- Sexual dysfunction, sweating

Life-threatening or Dangerous Side Effects
- Paralytic ileus, hyperthermia (TCAs + anticholinergic agents)
- Lowered seizure threshold and rare seizures
- Orthostatic hypotension, sudden death, arrhythmias, tachycardia
- QTc prolongation
- Hepatic failure, extrapyramidal symptoms
- Increased intraocular pressure, increased psychotic symptoms
- Rare induction of mania
- Rare activation of suicidality

Potential Advantages
- Less activating than stimulants
- For narcolepsy, may help patients who are insufficiently responsive to stimulants

Potential Disadvantages
- Has abuse potential
- Requires a second dose in the middle of the night

FIGURE 3.14. Prescribing information for tricyclic antidepressants (TCAs) (Stahl, 2014).

Prescribing Tips: SNRIs

Commonly Prescribed for *(bold for FDA-approved)*

- **Depression (venlafaxine, duloxetine)**
- **Generalized anxiety disorder (GAD) (venlafaxine, duloxetine)**
- **Social anxiety disorder (social phobia) (venlafaxine)**
- **Panic disorder (venlafaxine)**
- **Diabetic peripheral neuropathic pain (DPNP) (duloxetine)**
- **Fibromyalgia (duloxetine)**
- **Chronic musculoskeletal pain (duloxetine)**
- Stress urinary incontinence and neuropathic pain/chronic pain (duloxetine)
- Posttraumatic stress disorder (PTSD) and premenstrual dysphoric disorder (PMDD) (venlafaxine)

Usual Dosage Range

- Venlafaxine: 75–225 mg/day, once daily (ER) or divided into 2–3 doses (IR)
- Duloxetine: 40–60 mg/day in 1–2 doses

Dosage Forms

- Venlafaxine: capsule (ER): 37.5 mg, 75 mg, 150 mg; tablet (ER): 37.5 mg, 75 mg, 150 mg, 225 mg; tablet: 25 mg scored, 37.5 mg scored, 50 mg scored, 75 mg scored, 100 mg scored
- Duloxetine: capsule: 20 mg, 30 mg, 60 mg

How to Dose

- Varies depending on agent

Habit Forming

- No

Side Effects

- Nausea, diarrhea, decreased appetite, insomnia, sedation, sweating
- Sexual dysfunction
- Increase in blood pressure
- Dry mouth, constipation, dizziness, urinary retention (duloxetine)
- Headache, nervousness, asthenia, syndrome of inappropriate antidiuretic hormone secretion (SIADH), hyponatremia (venlafaxine)

Life-threatening or Dangerous Side Effects

- Rare seizures
- Rare induction of hypomania
- Rare activation of suicidality

Potential Advantages

- Patients with retarded or atypical depression
- Patients with comorbid anxiety
- Depressed patients with somatic symptoms, fatigue, and pain
- Patients with depression may have higher remission rates on SNRIs than on SSRIs

Potential Disadvantages

- Patients sensitive to nausea
- Patients with borderline or uncontrolled hypertension or cardiac disease (venlafaxine)
- Patients with urological disorders, prostate disorders (duloxetine)

FIGURE 3.15. Prescribing information for serotonin-norepinephrine reuptake inhibitors (SNRIs) (Stahl, 2014).

Prescribing Tips: Fluoxetine

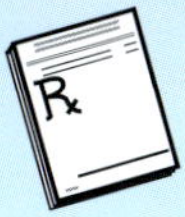

Commonly Prescribed for *(bold for FDA-approved)*
- **Major depressive disorder (MDD) (ages 8 and older)**
- **Obsessive compulsive disorder (OCD) (ages 7 and older)**
- **Premenstrual dysphoric disorder (PMDD)**
- **Bulimia nervosa**
- **Panic disorder**
- **Bipolar depression (in combination with olanzapine)**
- **Treatment-resistant depression (in combination with olanzapine)**
- Social anxiety disorder (social phobia)
- Posttraumatic stress disorder (PTSD)

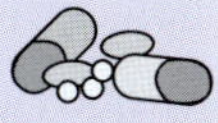

Usual Dosage Range
- 20–80 mg for depression and anxiety disorders

Dosage Forms
- Capsule: 10 mg, 20 mg, 40 mg, 60 mg
- Tablet: 10 mg
- Liquid: 20 mg/5 mL–120 mL bottles
- Weekly capsule: 90 mg

How to Dose
- Depression and OCD: initial dose 20 mg/day in the morning; usually wait a few weeks to assess drug effects before increasing dose; maximum dose generally 80 mg/day

Habit Forming
- No

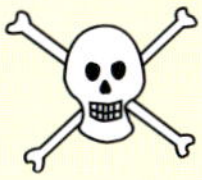

Side Effects
- Sexual dysfunction
- Gastrointestinal (decreased appetite, nausea, diarrhea, constipation, dry mouth)
- Mostly central nervous system (insomnia but also sedation, agitation, tremors, headache, dizziness)
- Autonomic (sweating)
- Bruising and rare bleeding

Life-threatening or Dangerous Side Effects
- Rare seizures
- Rare induction of mania
- Rare activation of suicidality

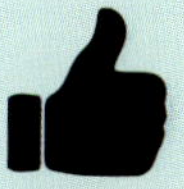

Potential Advantages
- Patients with atypical depression
- Patients with fatigue and low energy
- Patients with comorbid eating and affective disorders

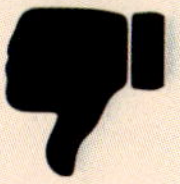

Potential Disadvantages
- Patients with anorexia
- Initiating treatment in anxious, agitated patients
- Initiating treatment in severe insomnia

FIGURE 3.16. Prescribing information for the selective serotonin reuptake inhibitor (SSRI) fluoxetine (Stahl, 2014).

Commonly Prescribed for *(bold for FDA-approved)*
- **Major depressive disorder (MDD) (transdermal)**
- **Parkinson's disease or symptomatic parkinsonism (oral, adjunctive)**
- Treatment-resistant depression
- Panic disorder (transdermal)
- Social anxiety disorder (transdermal)
- Treatment-resistant anxiety disorders (transdermal)
- Alzheimer's disease and other dementias (oral)

Usual Dosage Range
- Depression (transdermal): 6 mg/24 hours–12 mg/24 hours
- Depression (oral): 30–60 mg/day

Dosage Forms
- Transdermal patch: 20 mg/20 cm2 (6 mg/24 hours), 30 mg/30 cm2 (9 mg/24 hours), 40 mg/40 cm2 (12 mg/24 hours)
- Capsule: 5 mg
- Tablet: 5 mg scored
- Orally disintegrating tablet: 1.25 mg

How to Dose
- Depression (transdermal): initial dose 6 mg/24 hours; can increase by 3 mg/24 hours every 2 weeks; maximum dose generally 12 mg/24 hours

Habit Forming
- Lack of evidence for abuse potential with transdermal selegiline despite its metabolism to l-amphetamine and l-methamphetamine
- Some patients have developed dependence on other MAOIs

Side Effects
- Transdermal: application site reactions, headache, insomnia, diarrhea, dry mouth
- Oral: exacerbation of levodopa side effects, especially nausea, dizziness, abdominal pain, dry mouth, headache, dyskinesia, confusion, hallucinations, vivid dreams

Life-threatening or Dangerous Side Effects
- Transdermal: hypertensive crisis was not observed with preliminary experience in clinical trials, even in patients who were not following a low tyramine diet
- Oral: hypertensive crisis, especially when MAOIs are used with certain tryamine containing foods or prohibited drugs; reduced risk at low oral doses compared to nonselective MAOIs
- When used at high doses, may induce seizures and mania, as do nonselective MAOIs
- Rare activation of suicidality

Potential Advantages
- Treatment-resistant depression
- Patients with atypical depression
- Patients who wish to avoid weight gain and sexual dysfunction

Potential Disadvantages
- Noncompliant patients
- Patients with motor complications and fluctuations on levodopa treatment
- Patients with cardiac problems or hypertension

FIGURE 3.17. Prescribing information for the monoamine oxidase inhibitor (MAOI) selegiline (Stahl, 2014).

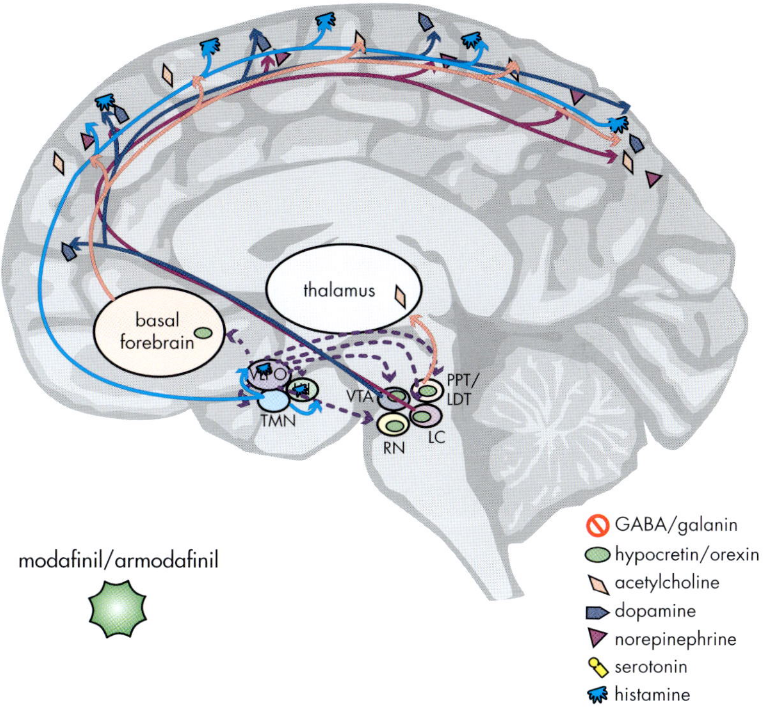

FIGURE 3.18. Although the exact mechanisms by which modafinil and its R-enantiomer, armodafinil, decrease sleep are not fully understood, evidence suggests that these agents promote wakefulness by acting directly or indirectly on many components of the sleep/wake circuit. Modafinil and armodafinil are hypothesized to inhibit GABA and promote dopamine, norepinephrine, histamine, and hypocretin/orexin (Morrissette, 2013).

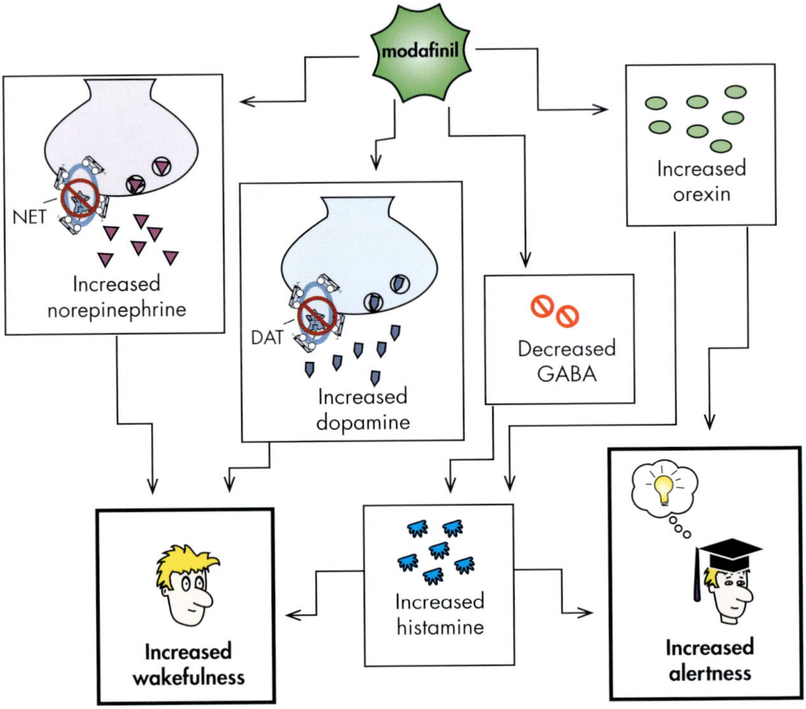

FIGURE 3.19. Modafinil and its R-enantiomer, armodafinil, increase both norepinephrine (NE) and dopamine (DA), possibly via their blockade of both the NE and DA reuptake transporters (NET and DAT, respectively). The actions of NE at alpha-adrenergic receptors and DA at dopamine D2 receptors are thought to contribute to the wake-promoting properties of modafinil. Orexin is a key component of the arousal system; thus, the hypothesized action of modafinil on the orexinergic system may help increase alertness. Additionally, modafinil may indirectly increase histamine, either by reducing GABAergic inhibition of histaminergic neurons or via actions at orexinergic neurons. The increase in histamine may contribute to both the wake-promoting effects of modafinil as well as the potential of modafinil to increase alertness (Morrissette, 2013).

Prescribing Tips: Modafinil/Armodafinil

Commonly Prescribed for *(bold for FDA-approved)*

- **Reducing excessive sleepiness in patients with narcolepsy and shift work**
- **sleep disorder**
- **Reducing excessive sleepiness in patients with obstructive sleep apnea/ hypopnea syndrome (OSAHS) (adjunct to standard treatment for underlying airway obstruction)**
- Attention deficit hyperactivity disorder (ADHD)
- Fatigue and sleepiness in depression
- Fatigue in multiple sclerosis
- Bipolar depression

Usual Dosage Range

- Modafinil: 200 mg/day in the morning
- Armodafinil: 150–250 mg/day

Dosage Forms

- Modafinil: tablet: 100 mg, 200 mg scored
- Armodafinil: tablet: 50 mg, 150 mg, 250 mg

How to Dose

- Modafinil: titration up or down only necessary if not optimally efficacious at the standard starting dose of 200 mg once a day in the morning
- Armodafinil: titration up or down only necessary if not optimally efficacious at the standard starting dose of 150 mg once a day
- For OSA and narcolepsy, give as a single dose in the morning
- For shift work sleep disorder, give as a single dose 1 hour prior to the start of the work shift

Habit Forming

- Schedule IV; may have some potential for abuse but unusual in clinical practice

Side Effects

- Headache
- Anxiety, nervousness, insomnia
- Dry mouth, diarrhea, nausea, anorexia
- Pharyngitis, rhinitis, infection
- Hypertension
- Palpitations

Life-threatening or Dangerous Side Effects

- Transient EKG ischemic changes in patients with mitral valve prolapse or left ventricular hypertrophy have been reported (rare)
- Rare activation of (hypo)mania, anxiety, hallucinations, or suicidal ideation
- Rare severe dermatological reactions (Stevens-Johnson syndrome and others)
- Angioedema, anaphylactoid reactions, and multi-organ hypersensitivity reactions have been reported

Potential Advantages

- Selective for areas of the brain involved in sleep/wake promotion
- Less activating and less abuse potential than stimulants

Potential Disadvantages

- May not work as well as stimulants in some patients

FIGURE 3.20. Prescribing information for the wake-promoting agent modafinil and its R-enantiomer, armodafinil (Stahl, 2014).

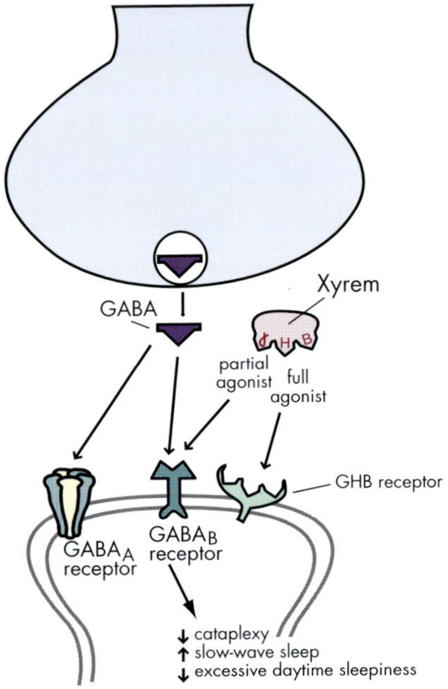

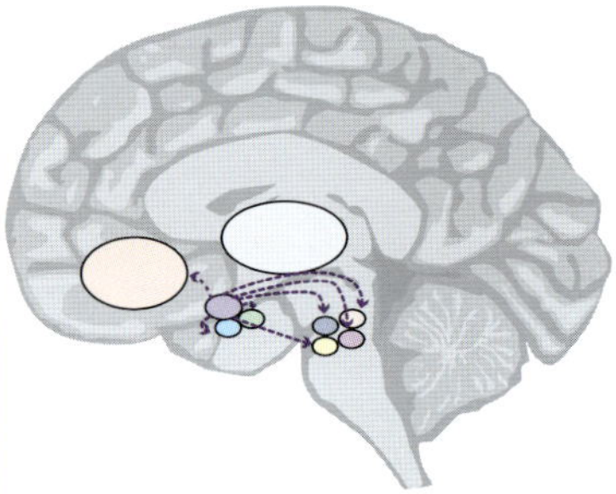

FIGURE 3.21. Sodium oxybate, also known as gamma-hydroxybutyrate (GHB), is a full agonist at gamma-hydroxybutyrate (GHB) receptors and a partial agonist at GABA-B receptors. As a GABA-B partial agonist, sodium oxybate acts as an antagonist when GABA levels are elevated and as an agonist when GABA levels are low. It is hypothesized that sodium oxybate increases slow-wave sleep and improves cataplexy via these actions at GABA-B receptors. Sodium oxybate is approved for use in both cataplexy and excessive sleepiness, and it appears to enhance slow-wave sleep and reduce hypnagogic hallucinations and sleep paralysis (Stahl, 2013; Hirai and Nishino, 2011; Adenuga and Attarian, 2014).

Prescribing Tips: Sodium Oxybate

Commonly Prescribed for *(bold for FDA-approved)*
- **Reducing excessive sleepiness in patients with narcolepsy**
- **Cataplexy in patients with narcolepsy**
- Fibromyalgia
- Chronic pain/neuropathic pain

Usual Dosage Range
- 6–9 g/night in 2 doses, 2.5–4 hours apart

Dosage Forms
- Oral solution: 500 mg/mL

How to Dose
- Initial dose 2.25 g at bedtime while seated in bed; second dose of 2.25 g should be taken 2.5–4 hours later, also while seated in bed; dosing can be increased by 1.5 g/night every 1–2 weeks

Habit Forming
- Medical use of sodium oxybate is classified under Schedule III
- Non-medical use of sodium oxybate is classified under Schedule I
- Some patients may develop dependence and/or tolerance; risk may be greater with higher doses
- History of drug addiction may increase risk of dependence

Side Effects
- Headache, dizziness, sedation
- Nausea, vomiting
- Enuresis

Life-threatening or Dangerous Side Effects
- Respiratory depression, especially when taken in overdose
- Neuropsychiatric events (psychosis, depression, paranoia, agitation)
- Confusion and wandering at night (unclear if this is true somnambulism)

Potential Advantages
- Less activating than stimulants
- For narcolepsy, may help patients who are insufficiently responsive to stimulants

Potential Disadvantages
- Has abuse potential
- Requires a second dose in the middle of the night

FIGURE 3.22. Prescribing information for sodium oxybate (Stahl, 2014).

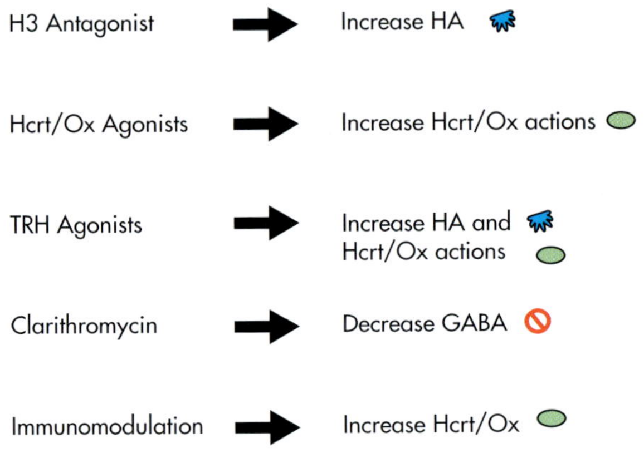

FIGURE 3.23. There are several agents currently being investigated for the treatment of hypersomnia. These include histamine H3 receptor antagonists, hypocretin/orexin (Hcrt/Ox) agonists, thyrotropin-releasing hormone (TRH) agonists, and the antibiotic clarithromycin. Additional treatment strategies include immunomodulation with immunoglobulins and blockade of T-cell entry into the brain. Antagonism of the histamine H3 receptor may increase histamine neurotransmission, leading to enhancement of the wake circuit (Stahl, 2013). Treatment with Hcrt/Ox agonists may be especially beneficial to patients with narcolepsy due to loss of Hcrt/Ox neurons; however, the development of an Hcrt/Ox agonist that readily crosses the blood-brain barrier has been unsuccessful so far (Adenuga and Attarian, 2014; Dauvilliers and Tafti, 2006; Hirai and Nishino, 2011; Mignot, 2012). Thyrotropin-releasing hormone (TRH) promotes histamine release from the tuberomammillary nucleus (TMN) and modulates Hcrt/Ox from the lateral hypothalamus (LH); therefore, TRH agonists may be effective in stimulating the wake circuitry on multiple levels (Gonzalez et al., 2009; Parmentier et al., 2009). Clarithromycin is an antibiotic that acts as a GABA-A receptor antagonist and may therefore reduce activation of the sleep circuit to promote wakefulness (Trotti et al., 2013; Trotti et al., 2015). Immunomodulation-based treatments seek to prevent the hypothesized autoimmune reaction that leads to the death of Hcrt/Ox (Dauvilliers et al., 2009; Knudsen et al., 2012).

4

Summary

As our understanding of the neurobiological and molecular bases of sleep expands, it is becoming increasingly clear that both the quality and quantity of sleep can greatly affect our physical and mental health; it is therefore critical that disorders of hypersomnolence be adequately recognized and appropriately managed. As the state of the science of sleep improves, so does our ability to differentially diagnose and effectively treat disorders of hypersomnolence such as narcolepsy. There are several treatment options available to effectively address symptoms of hypersomnia by targeting various components of the sleep/wake circuit, and there are several agents under investigation for their potential as treatments and possibly disease-modifying drugs for narcolepsy and other hypersomnias.

5 References

Adenuga O, Attarian H. Treatment of disorders of hypersomnolence. *Curr Treatment Options Neurol* 2014;16:302.

Ahmed I, Thorpy M. Clinical features, diagnosis and treatment of narcolepsy. *Clin Chest Med* 2010;31:371-81.

Bourgin P, Zeitzer JM, Mignot E. CSF hypocretin-1 assessment in sleep and neurological disorders. *Lancet Neurol* 2008;7(7):649-62.

Brancaccio M, Enoki R, Mazuski CN et al. Network-mediated encoding of circadian time: the suprachiasmatic nucleus (SCN) from genes to neurons to circuits, and back. *J Neurosci* 2014;34(46):15192-9.

Buysse DJ, Reynolds CF III, Monk TH et al. The Pittsburgh Sleep Quality Index: a new instrument for psychiatric practice and research. *Psychiatry Res* 1989;28(2):193-213.

Cappuccio FP et al. Sleep duration and all-cause mortality: a systematic review and meta-analysis of prospective studies. *Sleep* 2010;33(5):585-92.

Cermakian N, Lange T, Golombek D et al. Crosstalk between the circadian clock circuitry and the immune system. *Chronobiol Int* 2013;30(7):870-88.

Colwell CS. Linking neural activity and molecular oscillations in the SCN. *Nat Rev Neurosci* 2011;12(10):553-69.

Dauvilliers Y, Tafti M. Molecular genetics and treatment of narcolepsy. *Ann Med* 2006;38:252-62.

Dauvilliers Y, Abril B, Mas E et al. Normalization of hypocretin-1 in narcolepsy after intravenous immunoglobulin treatment. *Neurology* 2009;73(16):1333-4.

De la Herran-Arita, Garcia-Garcia F. Narcolepsy as an immune-mediated disease. *Sleep Disord* 2014; Epub ahead of print.

Dresler M, Spoormaker VI, Beitinger P et al. Neuroscience-driven discovery and development of sleep therapeutics. *Pharmacol Ther* 2014;141(3):300-34.

Froy O. Metabolism and circadian rhythms—implications for obesity. *Endocr Rev* 2010;31(1):1-24.

Golombek DA, Casiraghi LP, Agostino PV et al. The times they are a-changing: effects of circadian desynchronization on physiology and disease. *J Physiol* (Paris) 2013;107:310-22.

Guo X, Zheng L, Wang J et al. Epidemiological evidence for the link between sleep duration and high blood pressure: a systematic review and meta-analysis. *Sleep Med* 2013;14(4):324-32.

Harris J, Lack L, Kemo K et al. A randomized controlled trial of intensive sleep retraining (ISR): a brief conditioning treatment for chronic insomnia. *Sleep* 2012;35(1):49-60.

Hirai N, Nishino S. Recent advances in the treatment of narcolepsy. *Curr Treatment Options Neurol* 2011;13:437-57.

Knudsen S, Biering-Sørensen B, Kornum BR et al. Early IVIg treatment has no effect on post-H1N1 narcolepsy phenotype or hypocretin deficiency. *Neurology* 2012;79(1):102-3.

Krystal AD, Harsh JR, Yang R et al. A double-blind, placebo-controlled study of armodafinil for excessive sleepiness in patients with treated obstructive sleep apnea and comorbid depression. *J Clin Psychiatry* 2010;71(1):32-40.

Lallukka T, Kaikkonen R, Härkänen T et al. Sleep and sickness absence: a nationally representative register-based follow-up study. *Sleep* 2014;37(9):1413-25.

Larson-Prior LJ, Ju YE, Galvin JE. Cortical-subcortical interactions in hypersomnia disorders: mechanisms underlying cognitive and behavioral aspects of the sleep-wake cycle. *Frontiers Neurol* 2014;5(165): Epub ahead of print.

Liu Y et al. Sleep duration and chronic disease among US adults age 45 years and older: evidence from the 2010 behavioral risk factor surveillance system. *Sleep* 2013;36(10):1421-7.

Mahler SV et al. Motivational activation: a unifying hypothesis of orexin/hypocretin function. *Nat Neurosci* 2014;17(10):1298-1303.

Martin JL, Hakim AD. Wrist actigraphy. *Chest* 2011;139(6):1514-27.

Mignot EJM. A practical guide to the therapy of narcolepsy and hypersomnia syndromes. *Neurotherapeutics* 2012;9:739-52.

Morgenthaler TI, Kapur VK, Brown T et al. Practice parameters for the treatment of narcolepsy and other hypersomnias of central origin. *Sleep* 2007;30(12):1705-11.

Morrissette DA. Twisting the night away: a review of the neurobiology, genetics, diagnosis, and treatment of shift work disorder. *CNS Spectrums* 2013;18(suppl 1):45-53.

Ohayon MM. Determining the level of sleepiness in the American population and its correlates. *J Psychiatr Res* 2012;46:422-7.

Orzel-Gryglewska J. Consequences of sleep deprivation. 2010;23(1):95-114.

Palma JA, Urrestarazu E, Iriarte J. Sleep loss as a risk factor for neurologic disorders: a review. *Sleep Med* 2013;14(3):229-36.

Parmentier R, Kolbaev S, Klyuch BP et al. Excitation of histaminergic tuberomammillary neurons by thyrotropin-releasing hormone. *J Neurosci* 2009;29(14):4471-83.

Pigeon WR, Pinquart M, Conner K. Meta-analysis of sleep disturbance and suicidal thoughts and behaviors. *J Clin Psychiatry* 2012;73(9):e1160-7.

Reeve K, Bailes B. Insomnia in adults: etiology and management. *JNP* 2010;6(1):53-60.

Roth T, Roehrs T. Sleep organization and regulation. *Neurology* 2000;54(5 Suppl):S2-7.

Sangal RB, Thomas L, Mitler MM. Maintenance of wakefulness test and multiple sleep latency test. Measurement of different abilities in patients with sleep disorders. *Chest* 1992;101(4):898-902.

Sehgal A, Mignot E. Genetics of sleep and sleep disorders. *Cell* 2011;146(2):194-207.

Stahl SM. Stahl's essential psychopharmacology: neuroscientific basis and practical applications. 4th ed. New York, NY: *Cambridge University Press*; 2013.

Stahl SM. Stahl's essential psychopharmacology: the prescriber's guide. 5th ed. New York, NY: *Cambridge University Press*; 2014.

Stippig A, Hübers U, Emerich M. Apps in sleep medicine. *Sleep Breathing* 2015;19(1):411-7.

Tafti M. Genetic aspects of normal and disturbed sleep. *Sleep Med* 2009;10:S17-21.

Thaiss CA, Zeevi D, Levy M et al. Transkingdom control of microbiota diurnal oscillations promotes metabolic homeostasis. *Cell* 2014;159(3):514-29.

Thorpy MJ, Dauvilliers Y. Clinical and practical consideration in the pharmacologic management of narcolepsy. Sleep Med 2014; Epub ahead of print.

Trotti LM, Saini P, Bliwise DL et al. Clarithromycin in γ-aminobutyric acid-related hypersomnolence: a randomized, crossover trial. *Ann Neurol* 2015; Epub ahead of print.

Trotti LM, Saini P, Freeman AA et al. Improvement in daytime sleepiness with clarithromycin in patients with GABA-related hypersomnia: clinical experience. *J Psychopharmacol* 2013;28(7):697-702.

Van Someren EJ, Riemersma-Van Der Lek RF. Live to the rhythm, slave to the rhythm. *Sleep Med Rev* 2007;11(6):465-84.

Wulff K, Gatti S, Wettstein JG, Foster RG. Sleep and circadian rhythm disruption in psychiatric and neurodegenerative disease. *Nat Rev Neurosci* 2010;11(8):589-99.

Zaharna M, Dimitriu A, Guilleminault C. Expert opinion on pharmacotherapy of narcolepsy. *Expert Opinion Pharmacother* 2010;11(10):1633-45.

Zawilska JB, Skene DJ, Arendt J. Physiology and pharmacology of melatonin in relation to biological rhythms. *Pharmacol Rep* 2009;61(3):383-410.

Release/Expiration Dates

Print Monograph Released: October, 2015

Electronic Books Released: October, 2015

CME Credit Expires: October, 2018

CME Posttest Study Guide

The posttest questions have been provided below solely as a study tool to prepare for your online submission. ***NOTE: Posttests can only be submitted online. Faxed/mailed copies of the posttest cannot be processed*** *and will be returned to the sender. If you do not have access to a computer, contact customer service at 888-535-5600.*

1. Peter is a 34-year-old patient who complains of excessive daytime sleepiness that has persisted for over 3 years. As his clinician, you explain to Peter that diabetes, cardiovascular disease, and depression have all been associated with:

   A. Too much sleep
   B. Too little sleep
   C. Both too much sleep and too little sleep
   D. Neither too much sleep nor too little sleep

2. Which of the following statements regarding the suprachiasmatic nucleus (SCN) is most accurate?

   A. The dorsomedial shell contains cells that release the neuropeptides vasoactive intestinal peptide (VIP) and gastrin-releasing peptide (GRP)
   B. The ventrolateral core contains cells that release arginine vasopressin (AVP) and prokineticin 2 (PK2)
   C. The ventrolateral core receives the majority of the light coming through the retinohypothalamic tract
   D. All of the above
   E. None of the above

3. Which of the following actions are part of the sleep circuit:
    A. Histamine is released from the lateral hypothalamus
    B. Hypocretin/orexin is released from the tuberomammillary nucleus (TMN)
    C. Norepinephrine is released from the ventral tegmental area (VTA)
    D. GABA/galanin is released from the ventrolateral preoptic (VLPO) area
    E. All of the above
    F. None of the above

4. A 43-year-old woman with the autoimmune disorder lupus presents with excessive daytime sleepiness. The patient sometimes works the night shift as a nurse and is concerned that her ability to perform her job duties is being compromised by both her sleepiness and her lupus symptoms. You explain to the patient that job-related disturbance of her circadian rhythms and lupus symptoms could be related because there are many connections between sleep and immunity, including:
    A. Proinflammatory actions of melatonin at night
    B. Activation of the adaptive immune system at night
    C. Suppression of proinflammatory cytokines during the day
    D. Activation of the innate immune system during the day
    E. All of the above

5. Charles is a 27-year-old patient who complains of excessive daytime sleepiness. Further clinical assessment reveals that this patient does not feel refreshed upon waking and has a very short latency to sleep onset, despite typically sleeping 11 hours or more at night. Polysomnography indicates the absence of sleep onset REM periods (SOREMPs). Evaluation of the patient's cerebrospinal fluid (CSF) indicates that his hypocretin/orexin levels are within normal range but that his histamine levels are slightly lower than expected. After ruling out medical and psychiatric causes of hypersomnia for this patient, your most likely diagnosis would be:
    A. Idiopathic hypersomnia
    B. Kleine-Levin syndrome
    C. Narcolepsy with cataplexy
    D. Narcolepsy without cataplexy

6. Tina is a 31-year-old patient who complains of excessive sleepiness. She recently suffered injuries from a motor vehicle accident in which she fell asleep at the wheel. Clinical evaluation reveals cerebrospinal fluid (CSF) hypocretin/orexin levels within normal range and the presence of several sleep onset REM periods (SOREMPs) on polysomnography. After ruling out medical and psychiatric causes of hypersomnia for this patient, your most likely diagnosis would be:

   A. Narcolepsy with cataplexy
   B. Narcolepsy without cataplexy
   C. Idiopathic hypersomnia
   D. Kleine-Levin syndrome

7. An 11-year-old boy is brought in for evaluation by his concerned parents. The patient has recurrent periods of excessive sleepiness, despite sleeping for approximately 8 hours every night, accompanied by an insatiable appetite. His parents report that at times, the patient demonstrates reckless and disinhibited behavior; he was also recently suspended from school after his teacher found several adult magazines in his locker. Clinical evaluation reveals no medical or psychiatric causes of this behavior and hypocretin/orexin levels within normal range. Polysomnography indicates the absence of sleep onset REM periods (SOREMPs). Your most likely diagnosis for this patient would be:

   A. Idiopathic hypersomnia
   B. Narcolepsy with cataplexy
   C. Narcolepsy without cataplexy
   D. Kleine-Levin syndrome

8. Pharmacological strategies likely to promote wakefulness in patients with hypersomnia include:

   A. Increasing histaminergic neurotransmission
   B. Increasing orexinergic neurotransmission
   C. Decreasing histaminergic neurotransmission
   D. Decreasing orexinergic neurotransmission
   E. A and B
   F. B and C
   G. C and D

9. Michael is a 51-year-old patient who complains of excessive sleepiness. He drinks several cups of coffee and numerous energy drinks throughout the day in order to stay awake. Caffeine is believed to promote wakefulness by:

   A. Acting as an agonist at adenosine 2A receptors
   B. Acting as an antagonist at adenosine 2A receptors
   C. Acting as an agonist at dopamine D2 receptors
   D. Acting as an antagonist at dopamine D2 receptors

10. A 19-year-old woman with complaints of excessive daytime sleepiness, sleep paralysis, and loss of muscle tone when she laughs was recently diagnosed with narcolepsy with cataplexy. Which of the following is the only agent approved by the FDA for the treatment of both excessive sleepiness and cataplexy in narcolepsy?

   A. Modafinil
   B. Methylphenidate
   C. Fluoxetine
   D. Sodium oxybate
   E. Selegiline

CME Online Posttest and Certificate Instructions

There is no posttest fee nor fee for CME credits.

1. Read the book in sequence, evaluating the content presented
2. Complete the posttest and activity evaluation, available only online at www.neiglobal.com/CME (under "Book")
3. Print your certificate (if a score of 70% or more is achieved)
4. Questions? call 888-535-5600, or email CustomerService@NEIglobal.com